THE
EVERYTHING®
GUIDE TO
MACRONUTRIENTS

Dear Reader,

The world of nutrition is a tricky, deceiving, and downright confusing place. A quick search on the Internet or trip to the store reveals hundreds of different sources talking about the latest and greatest shortcut, magic pill, or weird trick for fat loss.

When you are looking to lose some weight and feel good about yourself, the number of diet plans you'll find is staggering. What is the one thing successful diets have in common? They help you reduce your calories without making you feel miserable. The successful diets are sustainable for life.

My goal with this book is to explain the truth about nutrition once and for all. After reading it, you'll know exactly how to eat to look good and remain healthy for the rest of your life. If you take the time to understand these principles and apply them to your individual goals, preferences, and lifestyle, you can get in the best shape of your life.

I truly believe this is the last diet book you'll ever need, and I hope you use it well.

To your health,

Matt Dustin

Welcome to the EVERYTHING® Series!

These handy, accessible books give you all you need to tackle a difficult project, gain a new hobby, comprehend a fascinating topic, prepare for an exam, or even brush up on something you learned back in school but have since forgotten.

You can choose to read an Everything® book from cover to cover or just pick out the information you want from our four useful boxes: e-questions, e-facts, e-alerts, and e-ssentials.

We give you everything you need to know on the subject, but throw in a lot of fun stuff along the way too.

We now have more than 400 Everything® books in print, spanning such wide-ranging categories as weddings, pregnancy, cooking, music instruction, foreign language, crafts, pets, New Age, and so much more. When you're done reading them all, you can finally say you know Everything®!

QUESTION

Answers to common questions

FACT

Important snippets of information

ALERT

Urgent warnings

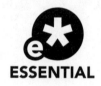

ESSENTIAL

Quick handy tips

PUBLISHER Karen Cooper

MANAGING EDITOR Lisa Laing

COPY CHIEF Casey Ebert

ASSISTANT PRODUCTION EDITOR Jo-Anne Duhamel

ACQUISITIONS EDITOR Zander Hatch

SENIOR DEVELOPMENT EDITOR Brett Palana-Shanahan

EVERYTHING® SERIES COVER DESIGNER Erin Alexander

Visit the entire Everything® series at www.everything.com

THE
EVERYTHING®
GUIDE TO
MACRONUTRIENTS

The flexible eating plan for losing fat and getting lean

Matt Dustin, CSCS, Pn1

Adams Media

New York London Toronto Sydney New Delhi

This book is dedicated to anyone who's ever felt confused,
discouraged, or frustrated when trying to understand nutrition. May this
book help you learn the truth about nutrition once and for all.

Aadamsmedia

Adams Media
An Imprint of Simon & Schuster, Inc.
57 Littlefield Street
Avon, Massachusetts 02322

An Everything® Series Book.
Everything® and everything.com® are registered trademarks of Simon & Schuster, Inc.

First Adams Media trade paperback edition NOVEMBER 2017

ADAMS MEDIA and colophon are trademarks of Simon and Schuster.

For information about special discounts for bulk purchases, please contact Simon & Schuster Special Sales at 1-866-506-1949 or business@simonandschuster.com.

The Simon & Schuster Speakers Bureau can bring authors to your live event. For more information or to book an event contact the Simon & Schuster Speakers Bureau at 1-866-248-3049 or visit our website at www.simonspeakers.com.

Manufactured in the United States of America

10 9 8 7 6 5 4 3

Library of Congress Cataloging-in-Publication Data
Dustin, Matt, author.
The everything guide to macronutrients / Matt Dustin, CSCS, Pn1.
Avon, Massachusetts: Adams Media, 2017.
Series: Everything.
Includes bibliographical references and index.
LCCN 2017026434 | ISBN 9781507204160 (pb) | ISBN 9781507204177 (ebook)
LCSH: Weight loss. | Carbohydrates. | Carbohydrates in human nutrition. | BISAC: COOKING / Health & Healing / General. | HEALTH & FITNESS / Diets. | HEALTH & FITNESS / General.
LCC RM222.2 .D787 2017 | DDC 641.5/6383--dc23
LC record available at https://lccn.loc.gov/2017026434

ISBN 978-1-5072-0416-0
ISBN 978-1-5072-0417-7 (ebook)

Contents

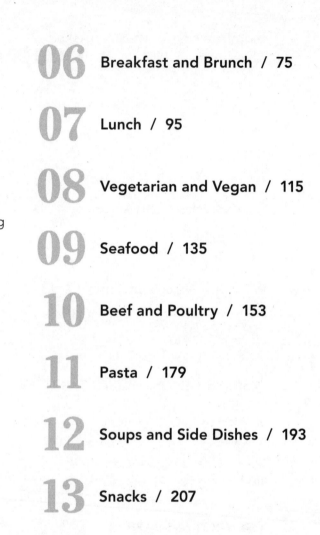

Acknowledgments

Without the support and encouragement of my friends and family as I've pursued my dreams of becoming a successful writer and fitness coach, this book wouldn't be possible. A special thank-you goes to Maria for putting up with me and always pushing me to keep going when things get tough.

Thank you to Zander Hatch and the rest of the fine folks at Simon & Schuster for bringing me back for a second book; you guys are the best. Lastly, thank you to John Romaniello for being a fantastic mentor and showing me what good writing looks like, and thank you to everyone else in the RFS group for helping me become a better writer, coach, and most importantly, a better human being.

Top 10 Benefits of the Macronutrient Diet

1. You can get in the best shape of your life while eating foods you love.

2. The diet adapts to your lifestyle and schedule.

3. There are no restrictive rules or requirements to carry around five small meals a day.

4. The macronutrient diet is not just a fat loss diet; it can be used by athletes, people trying to gain muscle, or just about anyone concerned with their overall health.

5. You can apply the principles of the macronutrient diet to any "style" of dieting, whether it's low-carb diets, low-fat diets, ketogenic diets, Paleo diets, or any other diet you can think of.

6. This diet is meant to be sustainable for life. It allows you to have a fun social life and still keep up with a healthy diet.

7. The diet teaches you how your individual body responds to various foods, something only you can figure out.

8. The macronutrient diet is the most accurate way to track and adjust your food intake so you can continue to make progress all the way to achieving your ideal body.

9. It can be fun building meal plans for yourself once you understand that no foods are completely off-limits.

10. The macronutrient diet builds self-control and teaches you to enjoy foods in moderation—a practice many tend to struggle with.

Introduction

THE MACRONUTRIENT DIET, ALSO known as flexible dieting or "If It Fits Your Macros" (IIFYM), is as useful as it is misunderstood.

Maybe you think that flexible dieting means you just eat junk food all day long that's carefully portioned. Maybe you think it means you'll have to carry a food scale around with you for the rest of your life, measuring and tracking every single thing you eat or drink. Neither of these are true.

The good news is that there is no strict approach to the macronutrient diet; no restrictive rules or limitations. Counting your macros is a way of tracking your food intake to ensure you're getting the right amounts of the right food for your body.

This diet requires more work than others, but it's also the most accurate and the most flexible diet. If you love pizza, cake, and wine, you can enjoy all of these things on a weekly basis. You just have to plan ahead and enjoy them in moderation. You'd be hard-pressed to find another diet that gives you permission to enjoy life the way a human being should.

If fitting in "junk" food isn't your thing, that's fine too. Flexible dieting simply refers to tracking your food and adjusting future consumption accordingly. The macronutrient diet is just as effective for the busy executive who wants to eat three meals a day and follow a low-carb diet as it is for the high-level athlete who's eating six small meals a day. This diet lends itself well to adapting to any special goals, needs, or dietary preferences.

This book should be the last diet book you ever need. Even if you read others after this book, you'll see how they, too, follow the principles you're about to learn. To lose fat, all you need to do is eat fewer calories than you need. Other strict diets do this by calling certain foods evil and restricting them completely. This restrictive approach works, but it's about as fun as getting a cavity filled.

Don't just read this book and put it back on the shelf. This diet requires work, there's no doubt about it. You'll be building your own meal plans completely tailored to your lifestyle, as well as tracking your food and having some self-control. It takes practice and patience as you learn how to track your food and eat for your needs. However, the end result is worth it. You'll learn how to get the body of your dreams, but that's just the tip of the iceberg. If you take the time to understand and apply this book, you'll understand the fundamental rules of nutrition, which is a skill that will serve you well for the rest of your life.

Read the book, work through the calculations, take the time to plan your meals and follow that plan, and you'll find dieting can actually be enjoyable. When you're following a diet built around foods you love, not a random diet you found in an old muscle magazine, you'll most likely find following that diet to be quite easy.

If you've tried every diet book without seeing the results you want, this book will finally help you get those results. There are no hidden secrets, insane rules, or secret hacks to your body. It takes an understanding of nutrition, a good plan, and execution. This book will help you understand and come up with that perfect plan. The execution is up to you.

Good luck.

CHAPTER 1

What Are Macronutrients?

Macronutrients are the building blocks of any diet—proteins, carbohydrates, and fats—and they are where all of your calories come from. Macronutrients supply the energy, fuel, and nutrients you need to live. Each macronutrient serves a specific purpose and should be consumed in the proper amount for optimal health. Quite a few variables come into play when setting up macronutrient ratios, but first, you must understand what they are, what they do, and what foods they come from.

Macronutrients Are the Building Blocks of Nutrition

Macronutrients form the basis of any nutrition plan. Regardless of whether you follow a strict diet plan or just eat whatever you feel like, you take in macronutrients every single day. Without an adequate macronutrient intake, your body would stop working. The amount of macronutrients in a given food determines how many calories are in that food. By figuring out exactly how many macronutrients your body needs each day and then eating just that balanced amount, you can achieve your health and weight loss goals.

ESSENTIAL

Macronutrients are proteins, carbs, and fat. An easy trick to remember this is remembering that macro means large. Micronutrients on the other hand, while essential, don't have any calories. Micronutrients would include vitamins, minerals, antioxidants, and other things found in food that don't have any calories.

To understand macronutrients, you need a very basic understanding of how your body operates. Every single process your body goes through every day, from brushing your teeth to digesting food and even breathing, requires energy. You may not feel physically tired from sitting on the couch watching television, but even the simple act of staying alive requires a little bit of energy. Your body gets the energy it needs from calories. Some foods have quite a few calories while some have very little, but all foods contain calories, even if they are found in very small amounts.

FACT

A calorie is a measure of energy. In scientific terms, a calorie is the amount of energy needed to increase the temperature of 1 kilogram of water by 1°C. Thus, the more calories a food contains, the more energy it supplies to your body. A calorie isn't "good" or "bad"—it just is. Different foods will offer more nutritional benefits than others, but ultimately a calorie is still a calorie and nothing more than a measure of energy.

If you have a very active lifestyle, your body will use or "burn" a greater number of calories to function every day. Activities that make you feel physically tired, like running, playing sports, yard work, or significant walking, will burn more calories than sitting around doing nothing.

Are Calories the Same As Fat?

The human body is very smart. It can survive without food for weeks at a time under extreme circumstances, and it's a very complex operating system. Your body uses energy every single day, but it also stores energy. Your body has a built-in storage system that allows it to save excess energy for a later time when you don't receive enough from food. Energy is stored in adipose cells, also known as body fat.

FACT

> There are two types of body fat: subcutaneous fat and visceral fat. Subcutaneous fat is found underneath the skin. Visceral fat is found deep within your body, mainly in the stomach area surrounding your internal organs. This deep belly fat is the dangerous kind; the kind that can have negative effects on important organs in your body.

That's right—that fat on your body contains stored energy, ready to be used when there isn't enough provided by the food you eat. Adipose tissue (body fat) provides some protection and insulation for your body, but at the end of the day, it's nothing more than stored energy.

Eating more calories does *not* necessarily cause fat gain. If you're an athlete or work a physical job, you need to be eating extra calories just to function.

The problem lies in excess calorie consumption. If you regularly eat more calories than your body burns in a day, that excess energy needs to go somewhere, and most of it will be stored as body fat. If you eat fewer calories than your body needs, you'll end up using some of your stored fat for energy, decreasing your body fat stores.

Later in this book, you'll learn all the details and calculations to figure out exactly how many calories you should be eating, but for now you just need to understand the basics of calories and body fat. At the end of the day, too many calories will lead to fat gain and too few will lead to fat loss. Fat loss has many intricacies and details, but at its most basic level, fat loss is nothing more than an energy equation.

ESSENTIAL

A quick and easy way to create a caloric deficit is to stop drinking liquid calories. Soft drinks, fruit juices, fancy coffee drinks—all of these can be loaded with calories that don't fill you up whatsoever. Your first order of business should be removing calorie-containing drinks from your diet, except for the occasional alcoholic drink.

Do You Need All Three?

Calories come from macronutrients, and there are three different macronutrients, or macros for short. They are protein, carbohydrates, and fats. Each of these macros play a unique role in how your body functions. If fat loss and body composition were a pyramid, total calories would form the base of that period, as that is the most important factor. However, the next level would be the actual quantities of macronutrients you consume each day.

You must have a proper balance of the three macros. Having too much or too little of any of the three will lead to less than optimal health and body functioning, as all three play important roles, and none of them are bad or evil. You'll learn to figure out your exact macronutrient needs later in this book, as the required levels of each will vary based on your goals.

It's worth mentioning that carbohydrates are the only nonessential macronutrient. You may feel miserable if you remove them completely from your diet, but assuming your protein and fat intake is correct, you won't suffer any dangerous side effects. If your protein or fat levels drop too low, you'll be looking at some real health problems, but you can live without carbohydrates. Removing them completely is an extreme form of dieting and not sustainable for most people, but it's a viable option if you really want to try it.

A Guide to Protein, Carbohydrates, and Fat

All calories come from the macronutrients found in food, which are carbohydrates, proteins, and fats. All of these macronutrients give you the calories you need to survive.

Carbohydrates: Fuel for Life

Carbohydrates, or carbs for short, come from starchy foods like potatoes and rice and some other fruits and vegetables. They are the body's preferred source of energy as they provide a quick form of energy. Where protein and fats are slow to digest, and not used as easily for energy, stored carbohydrates are very easy for your body to digest and use for energy. When you need a fast energy supply, you don't want to mess around with proteins and fats, which digest slowly. Every gram of carbohydrate contains four calories.

QUESTION

Is alcohol a carbohydrate?
A gram of alcohol has seven calories, but as it doesn't provide any nutrition or any significant protein, carbohydrates, or fat, it's considered an "empty calorie." It gets you closer to your daily calorie goal without providing any value. If you consume alcohol and want to still hit your calorie goal for the day, you'll have to take away some calories from your daily food intake, and you'll lose that nutritional value.

All carbohydrates are broken down into molecules of glucose or fructose, which are simple sugar molecules. Plain table sugar? That's a carbohydrate. So are oatmeal, potatoes, rice, cucumbers, fruit juices, and many other common foods. You may hear people talk about "good carbs" or "bad carbs," but at the end of the day, all carbohydrates end up in the same place.

Carbohydrates are broken down and stored throughout the body in the form of glycogen, mainly in the muscles and liver. Glycogen is a readily available fuel source for your body, particularly for high-intensity activities. If you're playing sports, exercising, or doing anything physically active, your body is most likely using stored glycogen to fuel those activities.

Protein: Building Blocks

Proteins are made up of amino acids, which are the building blocks of most of the cells in the human body. Without amino acids, you'd be unable to replace the skin cells you lose every day, grow hair and fingernails, or rebuild and repair damaged muscle tissue. Proteins are essential for optimal health and body functioning. Every gram of protein has four calories.

Protein comes from meat, fish, eggs, dairy products, and some lentils, such as soybeans. It's often consumed as a dietary supplement in powdered form, particularly among those who regularly exercise.

Fats: Essential for Life

Fat rounds out the trio of key macronutrients and, like protein, it is essential to live. The right kinds of fat support healthy joints, cellular health, heart health, brain functioning, mood, and a whole host of other functions in the body. Unlike carbohydrates and proteins, however, certain fats are less than stellar and should be avoided for the most part. Whereas carbs and proteins each have four calories per gram, fat has nine calories per gram.

QUESTION

Doesn't fat make me fat?
No. This is a very common belief because they share the same name, but this is not true. Dietary fat that you eat in your food is essential for your body in certain amounts. Adipose tissue, or body fat, is simply stored calories. While eating foods high in fat *can* result in excess adipose tissue, consuming dietary fat in the correct amounts will not make you fat.

Dietary fat is simply another form of energy and nutrition; it does not directly correlate at all to actual body fat. The right fats supply the body with energy, help it retain crucial vitamins that require fat for absorption, protect the organs, and encourage healthy skin and hair.

Should You Track Calories or Macros?

The unfortunate reality is that you're probably going to have to track your food intake at some point. When you're just getting started with a healthy eating plan, it may be enough to clean up your diet by eliminating soda, fast food, candy, and other foods that would typically be considered "bad."

This won't last forever. Eventually you're going to have to track and measure what you're eating, at least for a while. The closer you get to your goal weight, the harder it will be, and you'll really have to know exactly what's going in your body to continue making progress. With that being said, what should you be tracking? Calories or macros?

QUESTION

I've tried tracking my food on an app, and the macronutrients and calories don't add up. Where are the extra calories coming from?
With food labels, it's very common for manufacturers to round up a bit just to make the label look a little cleaner. For example, if a food has 24 grams of protein, that would equate to 96 calories, but they may just round up to 100 calories for that food. If you're paying attention to your total macro intake and using some sort of app to track your food, don't worry if the calories are slightly off.

Well, you already know that calories come from macros. By definition, if you are tracking your macronutrients, you'll always know exactly how many calories you've consumed that day. It doesn't go both ways, however, as tracking calories alone isn't going to show you the exact macronutrient breakdown you're consuming.

If you're just getting started with food tracking, start by simply tracking total calories. This is easier to learn, and it'll build a good habit of paying attention to what you eat and what's in your food. Once you have this down, you can move on to tracking the specific macros you're consuming.

FACT

It's important to care about your internal health and how you feel, not just how you look. You can dramatically change your body composition and reduce fat by cutting your caloric intake down, but this doesn't mean you're healthy on the inside. Vitamins and minerals are essential to your immune system, hair and skin health, brain functioning, heart health, energy levels, and so many other important things.

Macronutrients versus Micronutrients

You may be wondering, if macros are proteins, carbohydrates, and fats, where do are all of those vitamins and minerals come from? Surely those are important?

The important nutritional value your food provides comes from micronutrients. These are the vitamins and minerals that allow your body to function at an optimal level. They are only required in small amounts, which is why they are called micronutrients, but they are very important.

Your body is capable of hundreds of internal functions, with many of them happening simultaneously. Even something as simple as breathing requires the coordinated efforts of several different systems and muscles in your body.

If you are missing micronutrients in your diet, your health will suffer. Vitamins and minerals are essential for proper growth, energy levels, metabolism, and a whole host of other functions. For optimal health levels, you should be consuming a wide variety of micronutrients in your diet every single day.

Nutrient-dense foods are the ones that provide the most nutritional value and should be a main staple of your diet. Foods like fruits, vegetables, lean proteins, whole grains, and healthy fats are all necessary to ensure you're getting the vitamins and minerals your body needs to run at 100 percent efficiency.

While it's possible to change your body composition with any sort of food you'd like, assuming the calories add up, your overall health is far more important than the number on the scale. You may think you're cheating the system if you try to get all of your daily calories from foods that are lacking in micronutrients, but this isn't ideal if you care about your long-term health.

Essential Micronutrients

Now that you know you need vitamins and minerals, it's time to look at what food sources supply them. There are many vitamins and minerals, so your best bet is to try and get a variety of fruits and vegetables every day and opt for whole, unprocessed foods whenever you can. Think the meat, eggs, and produce sections, not the packaged stuff in the middle aisles of the supermarket.

While covering every single vitamin and mineral and where it comes from is beyond the scope of this book, it's important to highlight some of the more important ones. The following seven micronutrients are some of the more important vitamins and minerals that play a massive role in staying healthy, and you should try to get them in your diet every single day.

The last thing to mention is the importance of using whole foods to meet your micronutrient goals rather than relying solely on supplements. While there are many different supplements on the market that offer vitamin and mineral support, nothing beats the nutritional value of whole foods. Supplements can be a good safety net, but if that's your only source of these micros, you're not going to see the full benefit of consuming them. Whole foods contain natural combinations of these vitamins and minerals so they can work together in your body to be even more effective, which is a benefit individual supplements are unable to replicate.

Vitamin D

Vitamin D is the sunshine vitamin and is most commonly associated with mood and happiness. It's produced when your skin is exposed to sunlight on a regular basis, and a deficiency in vitamin D can lead to weak bones, depression, mood swings, rickets, cardiovascular problems, and many more issues. Although our bodies can produce vitamin D naturally, direct exposure to sunlight on a daily basis is required to initiate the natural production process, something many people don't get enough of.

The best food sources for vitamin D are fatty fish, egg yolks, foods fortified with added vitamin D, or a supplement. If you are going to take a vitamin

D supplement, be sure to check with your doctor first to figure out the right dosage for you as it's a fat-soluble vitamin that can accumulate in your system if you take more than your body can process.

Vitamin C

Vitamin C is one that almost everybody knows as the immune system booster. When you start to get sick, you take extra vitamin C. While taking extra vitamin C when you're feeling under the weather can help strengthen your immune system, it's important to make sure you're getting enough even on the days when you aren't feeling sick. A lack of vitamin C has been linked to scurvy, a weak immune system, the tendency to bruise easily, and joint and muscle pain.

You can get vitamin C from oranges, kiwis, pineapple, papaya, kale, and various peppers. Eating a wide variety of fruits and vegetables every day is a good way to make sure you're getting plenty of this essential vitamin.

Vitamin B

There are several different types of vitamin B, but they all do the same thing. These are water-soluble vitamins, which means they can be absorbed and utilized without relying on dietary fat.

B vitamins help with cellular metabolism. They assist your body in absorbing the food you eat and using it for energy. These vitamins are also important for the formation of red blood cells, which transport oxygen to the various parts of your body.

You can supplement with vitamin B complexes or you can obtain them from whole-food proteins like meat, fish, eggs, and leafy green vegetables.

Vitamin K

Vitamin K is another fat-soluble vitamin that must be consumed with some dietary fat for your body to absorb it. Its most important role is in aiding with the formation of blood clots. If you cut yourself, you want your blood to form a clot as quickly as possible to stop the bleeding—a deficiency in vitamin K will make this very difficult.

Foods high in vitamin K include spinach, asparagus, broccoli, lentils, eggs, and meats. If you're eating a well-rounded diet that includes a variety of fruits and vegetables, you're probably getting enough vitamin K. If you don't eat many vegetables, you might want to consider eating more or supplementing with vitamin K.

Magnesium

Magnesium is a mineral found in dark leafy greens like spinach and kale, in addition to certain nuts. As researchers are learning more about this mineral, it's becoming quite clear that it's one of the most important minerals you can consume, and magnesium deficiency is becoming a dangerous epidemic.

Most leafy greens used to be very high in magnesium, but as modern farming methods have changed, the nutritional content of plants has started to decline. Magnesium deficiency can cause muscle cramping, muscle spasms, hormonal issues, high blood pressure, mood swings and depression, anxiety, lack of energy, and problems sleeping. It's extremely important to consume optimal levels of magnesium, and unless you are eating a lot of leafy greens every day, a supplement may be beneficial as a nutritional insurance.

Potassium

Potassium is an electrolyte, which is a mineral that helps your body send signals through the muscles. Without adequate potassium, your body's nerves may not function properly, and you may experience muscle cramping or twitching and have difficulty contracting your muscles the proper way. Because your body loses electrolytes when you sweat, it's important to get plenty of potassium in your diet if you lead an active life.

It is possible to have too much potassium, but a healthy liver will remove any excess potassium from your blood. Eating potassium-rich foods like bananas, spinach, squash, and avocados is the best way to ensure you are getting enough from natural food sources. If you tend to sweat a lot and notice muscle cramps during exercise, you may want to consume an electrolyte drink during your workouts to stay hydrated.

Calcium

Of all the minerals found in your body, calcium is the one you have in the greatest abundance, and up to 99 percent of it is stored in your bones and teeth. Beyond supporting a strong skeletal system, calcium also plays an important role in blood vessel and muscular contractions, as well as in the production of certain hormones and enzymes.

Calcium is primarily found in dairy products, so including milk, yogurt, and cheese in your diet is a good way to make sure you're getting enough calcium. It's also found in some dark leafy greens and can be supplemented if you follow a vegan diet that doesn't allow any dairy product intake.

CHAPTER 2

The Big Three

Just as all foods are not created equal, all macros are not created equal. This chapter will give you an in-depth look at proteins, carbohydrates, and fats, showing you what your best choices are in each macronutrient category. This chapter will also debunk a few common macronutrient myths and illuminate how some other restrictive diets can actually hurt your body while flexible eating allows you to keep your systems in proper working order. Having a better understanding of each macronutrient will allow you to make the best choices for your health and diet goals.

Simple versus Complex Carbs

You've probably heard of simple carbs and complex carbs. This simply refers to the speed at which they are broken down, digested, and absorbed into your bloodstream. Simple carbs are fast-digesting and complex carbs are slow-digesting.

ALERT

Carbohydrates often contain fiber. Fiber is very important for heart health, digestion, and controlling blood sugar. Foods that are higher in fiber will take longer to digest and will generally keep you full longer. The exact ranges vary from person to person based on factors like age, gender, and weight, but most people should aim to consume 25–40 grams of fiber per day.

Digestion speed is measured by something called the *glycemic index*. This is a complicated test, but it involves checking blood sugar levels, consuming carbohydrates, and then timing how long it takes to see an increase in blood sugar. All you need to know is that high-glycemic carbs are the ones that digest quickly and low-glycemic carbs digest a bit more slowly.

High-glycemic carbs come from foods like fruit, rice, candy, soda, juice, and any other "sugary" carb. They digest quickly and give you a quick hit of energy. Low-glycemic carbs come from whole grains, vegetables, and any carbohydrate that's a bit slow to digest. These typically take longer to break down, so you'll feel full longer and have a steady, slow release of energy.

FACT

Fiber absorbs water, which you've probably noticed if you've ever made oatmeal. When you consume high-fiber foods, they will tend to absorb the water in your body and can cause cramping or an upset stomach. Be sure to drink plenty of water to avoid any stomach discomfort from your fiber intake.

Carbs are unique in that they are the only nonessential macronutrient. If you don't get adequate levels of the other two macros, protein and fat, you could face serious health consequences. However, the human body can survive without any carbohydrate intake. If you ever hear that low-carb diets are dangerous or bad for your brain, this simply isn't true. Your body can turn fats and proteins into glucose if it needs to, but it can't turn carbs into fats and proteins.

FACT

The human body can take protein and fat molecules and convert them into glucose, which is what carbohydrates are made of. It's a slow process and less efficient than simply eating carbohydrates, but it can provide the body with glucose in the absence of dietary carbs. This process is called *gluconeogenesis*: the creation of new glucose.

Do "Bad Carbs" Exist?

Typically when someone talks about "bad carbs," they are referring to sugary, processed carb sources. These are things like candy, soda, fruit juice, or just about anything else that's sweet, delicious, and comes from a box.

The truth is, all carbohydrates are made up of simple sugar molecules. When fully broken down by your body's digestive system, carbohydrates are made up of either glucose or fructose, two simple sugar molecules. It doesn't matter if you get 40 grams of carbs from cake or from brown rice; your body reacts to the 40 grams of carbs.

Many popular diets preach the dangers of too much sugar. It's not a good idea to eat pure sugar, of course, but it really isn't as bad as the media would have you believe. Will drinking soda, a high-glycemic, fast-digesting carb, cause a blood sugar spike? Absolutely. The aftermath of that spike can leave you feeling hungry, moody, and tired.

Do you know what other foods supply fast-digesting, high-glycemic carbohydrates? White rice, bananas, kiwis, oranges…and the list goes on. Here's the difference: whole foods will be significantly higher in micronutrients, which are the vitamins and minerals you need to stay healthy. You'll get those in high quantities from fresh fruit and vegetables, and you'll get virtually none from processed sweets.

In terms of pure body composition, the carb source doesn't really matter. It's important to know this so that you don't associate desserts, soda, or any other carbs you enjoy with guilt and immediate fat gain.

For optimal health, you should be getting your carbs from whole foods. However, the occasional treat, assuming it fits into your daily calorie allotment, isn't going to derail your progress. It's much better to allow yourself to enjoy these treats in moderation if it helps you stay on track, rather than attempt to eliminate them completely and end up binge eating a whole cake on the weekend. Don't make a habit of getting all of your carbs from cookies, but understand that those cookies are not bad in and of themselves.

To help you plan your diet, here is a list of whole foods that contain primarily carbohydrates. Some foods will contain high amounts of multiple macronutrients, but these foods are mostly carbs. There will be similar lists for proteins and fats as well. The best way to learn what macros are in what foods is to start checking the nutritional information labels of the foods you buy, but the following lists will give you a quick reference guide to look at.

CARBOHYDRATE SOURCES
- Rice
- Oatmeal
- Pasta
- Fruit
- Bread
- Potatoes
- Squash

All Proteins Are Not Created Equal

Just like carbohydrates are classified as simple or complex, proteins also come in two varieties: complete and incomplete. Remember how proteins are made up of amino acids? Well, of those amino acids, nine are referred to as essential amino acids. Essential amino acids cannot be produced by the human body and must be obtained through food or supplements.

Protein is what allows you to rebuild your body and recover from the daily wear and tear you place on it. Often people associate high protein intake with gaining muscle, but that's just one role protein plays in the body. Every day, your body is regenerating hair, skin, fingernails, and yes, muscle tissue. It uses amino acids to do this, so if you aren't consuming enough from your diet, your body will start to rip apart and break down your muscle tissue to get those amino acids.

FACT

In terms of digestion, there is something called the *thermic effect of food*. Remember how every process in your body requires energy? Digestion is no different. Every food you eat requires some energy to break it down, absorb it, and put it to use or store for later. Protein has a high thermic effect, which means it burns quite a few calories simply from digesting it. You shouldn't try to adjust the total calorie content based on this, but it's good to know.

The other main benefit of protein is its ability to keep you feeling full. Whole-food protein sources are tough for your body to digest. This means that when you consume protein sources like meat, fish, or eggs, it's going to take your body longer to break them down compared to foods that consist of simple carbohydrates. If fat loss is your goal, increasing your protein intake is a fantastic way to keep yourself feeling full throughout the day, making your diet easier and preventing muscle breakdown as your food intake gets lower and lower.

If a protein source contains all nine essential amino acids, it's considered a complete protein. If it's lacking any of the essential amino acids, it's considered an incomplete protein. It's important that you get plenty of complete proteins throughout the day, whatever your diet of choice may be.

It's possible to supplement with amino acids, and many companies produce "branched-chain" or essential amino acid supplements. It's still better to get these amino acids from whole-food sources, but if you find you are struggling to get enough protein in your diet, an inexpensive essential amino acid supplement could help.

If you're a vegan or vegetarian, you still need complete proteins if you want to live a healthy life. Unfortunately, most plant-based proteins just aren't complete. Soy protein is one of the few complete plant proteins available, but excess soy consumption can have negative side effects, so try not to go overboard with the soy protein. If you follow a vegan diet, especially if you are active, you should strongly consider investing in a plant-based protein supplement to ensure you are reaching your daily goals.

Protein Myths

There are quite a few myths about protein, most of which are false. It's very important that you understand how important this nutrient is, so let's get to the bottom of things.

A common myth is that protein makes you bulky and should only be consumed by those who want to grow big, strong muscles. This simply isn't true. The process of growing new muscle is called *muscular hypertrophy*, and this occurs with regular resistance training such as body weight training or weight lifting. There's no need to fear protein intake, because you're never going to accidentally get too muscular.

QUESTION

What actually causes you to grow new muscle?
While protein plays a role in muscle growth, it's only a small part of the picture. Muscle growth, or hypertrophy, is the combined result of heavy resistance training that's performed consistently over a long period of time and excess caloric intake. If you're eating more than you need, getting adequate protein, and training your muscles with the appropriate intensity, you'll slowly start to gain more muscle.

You may have heard that eating too much protein or using protein supplements will damage your kidneys. This simply isn't true. Your body has to work harder to break down protein, but if anything, this is a good thing. Even at doses as high as 2 grams per pound of body weight (which is far more than anyone needs), protein intake is very safe.

PROTEIN SOURCES
- Chicken
- Turkey
- Beef
- Fish
- Dairy products
- Eggs
- Protein powder

Why You Need Fat to Live

Contrary to common belief, fat is not evil. The word itself sounds bad because it's often associated with body fat, which many people want to lose. The truth is, you *need* dietary fat for your body to function. There are good fats and bad fats, and some are better than others, but without adequate fat intake, you'll run into all sorts of health problems.

First, let's define body fat and dietary fat. When you talk about body fat, the stuff you probably want to lose, you're actually referring to what's known as *adipose tissue*. Adipose tissue contains adipose cells, which are storage units for energy.

If your diet provides more calories than you are able to burn, you'll store those calories in fat cells, causing you to store more body fat. Keep in mind that dietary fat intake does not cause body fat gain; excess calories from any macronutrient causes body fat gain. Dietary fat is simply another source of energy, just like proteins and carbs. Body fat is extra energy stored for later, but it can come from *any* food. Eating fat does not automatically make you fat.

There are several very important functions of dietary fats. In addition to being a good source of sustained, slow-releasing energy, they help support your cellular health and functioning. Without proper fat intake, many of the cells in your body wouldn't be able to operate at 100 percent efficiency. Certain essential nutrients, like vitamins A, D, E, and K, are fat-soluble, which means they can't be absorbed by your body without enough fat intake. If you take these vitamins or find them in foods that don't include some fat, your body won't be able to absorb and use them properly, and you may run into deficiencies.

The last important function of dietary fat is hormonal support. Fat supplies cholesterol, which is generally classified as HDL or LDL cholesterol. Too much cholesterol, particularly too much LDL cholesterol, can cause plaque formation and buildup in your heart. However, not getting enough cholesterol is also bad. Cholesterol is important for producing many hormones in the body, including important reproductive hormones, which is why those who follow very low-fat diets often report negative hormonal changes after a while. There's no need to go overboard with fat, but don't be afraid of including the right fats in your diet.

Good Fats and Bad Fats

In terms of dietary fat, there are several different kinds. The exact science of how they are classified is not necessary to know; just know that unsaturated fats are the best, saturated fats are decent, and trans fats should be avoided whenever possible. You also have monounsaturated fats and polyunsaturated fats, but the easiest thing is just to remember which foods provide the "good" fats—there will be a list later on in this section for you to reference.

ALERT

Avoid trans fats whenever possible. There are a few different types of fats, classified based on their molecular structure. They are unsaturated fats, saturated fats, and trans fats. Generally speaking, unsaturated fats and some saturated fats, which are found in avocados, egg yolks, red meat, nuts, coconut, and fish, are the "good fats." Trans fats, on the other hand, have been associated with a higher risk of heart disease and other negative effects. They are often found in fried and heavily processed foods.

The best sort of fat you can get is one that's high in omega-3 fatty acids. There are two common omegas: omega-3 fatty acids and omega-6 fatty acids. Omega-3s are found in fatty cuts of fish, egg yolks, avocados, and nuts, as well as a few other foods, and they can also be supplemented. Foods that are high in omega-3s are considered to be good fats.

Omega-6 fatty acids are very common in processed and fried foods like salad dressings, pizza, french fries, and sausages, in addition to certain cooking oils, such as vegetable oil. Omega-6 fatty acids are a tricky subject. They are essential, in that your body needs them and cannot produce them, but it's important to have the right balance between omega-6 and omega-3 fatty acids.

FACT

Omega-3 fatty acids have been associated with a very long list of health benefits, beyond simply providing a balance with omega-6s. They have been associated with increased mental function and focus, improved mood, decreased inflammation and joint pain, decreased risk of cardiovascular disease, improved insulin sensitivity for easier fat loss, and many more benefits. If you don't eat fatty cuts of wild-caught fish on a regular basis, you may want to consider using a daily fish oil supplement.

It's very common to have a diet that's much higher in omega-6s, as people tend to eat a lot of processed vending machine snacks and fast food. If your omega-6 fatty acid intake outweighs your omega-3 intake, you'll run into health problems, like increased inflammation and increased risk of cardiovascular disease. To get as close to a one-to-one ratio of omega-6 and omega-3 fatty acids as possible, be sure to eat plenty of good fats on a regular basis.

FAT SOURCES
- Egg yolks
- Avocado
- Nuts
- Coconut oil
- Red meat
- Fatty cuts of fish
- Cooking oils such as olive oil and macadamia nut oil

Balancing Macronutrients for Optimal Health

A healthy diet will consist of a balance of all three macronutrients. The most commonly recommended ratio is 40 percent protein, 40 percent carbohydrates, and 20 percent fat. Later chapters will detail exactly how to calculate your exact ratios based on your goals and lifestyle factors, but these numbers are a good general recommendation.

The total number of calories in your diet are determined by your macronutrient intake. If you decrease your total calorie intake, all of your macronutrient numbers will decrease as well. For a healthy, safe approach to weight loss, you should keep a balance of all three nutrients in your diet, rather than eliminating one altogether.

ESSENTIAL

If healthy weight loss is your goal, you shouldn't lose any more than 1 percent of your total body weight per week. For most people this ends up being right around 1–2 pounds per week. You may lose more in the beginning, but the healthiest approach is a slow and steady one. Losing weight too quickly is not healthy or sustainable.

If your goal is to lose body fat, you need to maintain a caloric deficit. You can do this by reducing your food intake or burning more calories through exercise, but without this deficit, fat loss will not happen. There is no magic pill or one evil food you can eliminate to instantly lose fat, no matter what magazine covers may claim. If you are trying to gain weight, you simply need to eat more calories than your body needs.

Some of the more common diet strategies can have negative side effects and aren't optimal for a healthy, sustainable body change. Always remember that any changes you make to your diet should be sustainable, lasting, and healthy, not short-term fixes that set you up to gain all of your weight back as soon as you stop the diet.

Low-Carb Diets

One of the most common diets is the low-carb or even zero-carb diet. You already know that carbohydrates are not essential to live, so if this diet is followed correctly, it wouldn't have any serious health consequences. However, for most people, it just isn't realistic to give up carbs completely for any long period of time. You'll have to eat extra fats to make up for those lost calories, and unless you're careful, it's easy to eat too much of the wrong sorts of fats and end up with health issues down the road.

Unless you are following a carb-cycling diet, which is not necessary and is a bit more advanced, it's probably best to avoid low-carb diets. It's not an unhealthy option and in theory it makes sense. However, giving up carbohydrates for good just isn't realistic for most people, and it would be more beneficial to learn to follow a balanced diet.

FACT

For every gram of glycogen your body stores, it also stores 3 grams of water. This means that if you remove carbohydrates from your diet completely, you'll drop a lot of water weight from your muscle and liver cells. Don't confuse this for fat loss if you follow a low-carb diet; that initial weight drop is mostly water. This works both ways; if you eat a high-carbohydrate meal, you'll hold excess water. No need to panic if the scale jumps overnight.

Low-Fat Diets

This type of diet is the one with the most potential to do more harm than good. Many people used to think that dietary fat was what caused fat gain, which remains a common misconception. You know the truth now, that excess calories are to blame and fats are okay.

When your fat intake drops too low, your hormonal levels will suffer. Hormones, particularly reproductive hormones, are dependent on fat. For both men and women, removing too much fat from a diet can lead to decreased energy, mood swings, and a decreased sex drive. Women often report irregular menstrual cycles as well when dietary fat intake drops too low.

Even if weight loss is your primary goal, you should still be concerned with your overall health first and foremost. Cutting out fat may help you lose weight, but it's probably going to have some serious negative side effects.

You don't need to go overboard and eat all the fat in sight, but you shouldn't eliminate it completely either. Moderation is key.

Healthy Choices in Theory and Practice

In a perfect world, all of your food would come from fresh, whole-food sources and supply perfectly balanced nutrition. In the real world, this simply isn't realistic for most people. Life is meant to be enjoyed, and you shouldn't have to make yourself miserable or become obsessed with your food choices to be healthy and maintain the body you want.

Most people find they are able to manage their nutrition while still enjoying themselves by following the $^{80}/_{20}$ rule of nutrition. This means that 80 percent of the time you choose healthy food sources to the best of your ability. The other 20 percent of the time you enjoy what would traditionally be considered "bad" foods—your favorite dessert, a few drinks, or a slice of pizza, for example.

If you can learn to fit those indulgences into your daily macronutrients without losing control and binge eating an entire pizza in one sitting, you'll find you can enjoy the foods you love on a regular basis and still see fantastic results.

The next chapters will go very in-depth on this topic and teach you the ins and outs of what foods to choose, why to choose them, how to build a meal plan suited to your lifestyle, and much more. It may require some practice and trial and error, but if you have some dedication and self-control, it's absolutely possible for anyone to enjoy the foods they love guilt-free and still work toward the healthy body they want to have.

CHAPTER 3

The Advantages of the Macronutrient Diet

There are many different diet plans available, and with so many to choose from, it's important to choose the one that's a good fit for your individual lifestyle and preferences. The macronutrient diet is easily adaptable to any dietary schedule, lifestyle, and preference. This chapter will take you through both the science of the macronutrient diet and also the wide range of benefits that this flexible diet offers. You'll also learn about your body's different energy burning cycles and how properly integrating your macronutrients throughout the day can help your progress.

The Science Behind the Diet

The macronutrient diet doesn't always make sense. After all, you've probably been told your entire life that you can only lose weight eating "clean" foods. Candy bars and pizza? Those foods make you fat. If you want to lose weight, you can only eat grilled chicken, sweet potatoes, egg whites, spinach, and asparagus.

This information is well-meaning—most of the time. A lot of so-called experts truly believe that you must eat these clean food sources if you want to lose weight and get healthy. This book isn't trying to show that eating indulgent foods is bad, not by any means. A diet full of whole foods is going to have significantly more nutritional benefit than a diet full of processed and packaged foods.

FACT

The macronutrient diet does not *require* you to eat junk food on a regular basis; it simply allows it. The macro diet, or flexible diet, simply refers to tracking your food, being precise with your macronutrient intake, and giving yourself the freedom to choose what foods you want to eat. Flexible dieting could be applied to carb cycling, a clean eating diet, the Paleo diet, a ketogenic diet, or any other diet really.

You must understand that the "clean eating" diet isn't the *only* way. It's very possible, and in fact more sustainable in the long term, to eat the foods you enjoy in moderation on a regular basis. The idea of giving up any one food forever is a scary idea, but if you know you can enjoy your favorite foods whenever you want, guilt-free, so long as you account for them, it makes the prospect of long-term dieting much easier.

Macronutrients and Energy

As you'll recall from Chapter 1, a calorie is simply a measure of energy, excess calories are stored as body fat, and calories come from protein, carbohydrates, and fat. That's a good basic understanding, but it's time to get a little more in-depth with that and look at the various ways your body uses energy and which macronutrients support those energy systems. The idea that excess calories will be stored for later usage is the big picture; now it's time to look at the details.

There are three categories of energy systems in your body—complex processes that produce the required energy for whatever activity you're doing. Within these categories are various subcategories, but unless you're concerned with elite levels of human performance optimization, the subcategories aren't particularly important to understand. For fat loss and nutrition, you just need to know the basics of the big three systems.

ESSENTIAL

It's very important to look at exercise as a means of improving your body's health—because it is. If you see it as punishment or strictly as a way to burn calories, it will be much harder to enjoy it and make it a sustainable habit. Remember, you are getting stronger and setting yourself up to live a longer, healthier life. Burning extra calories is just a nice side effect.

Whether you're sleeping in bed or sprinting up a hill, one of the three energy systems is at work. The scientific names for these systems are the ATP-PC system, glycolytic system, and oxidative system, but just think of them as the fast, medium, and slow energy systems.

The Fast Energy System (ATP-PC System)

This fast energy system is your maximum effort, short-duration system. It can supply an intense burst of energy for around 10–12 seconds before it runs out of steam and the next system takes over. This is used when you are jumping, lifting something very heavy, or doing a fast and short run, like sprinting across a basketball court.

In terms of nutrition, you don't really need to worry about this one too much. Just know it exists. Because it's such a short burst of energy, it uses something called *adenosine triphosphate* (ATP), which is made and stored in your muscle cells. As long as you're getting enough calories and nutrients, you'll have plenty of ATP available.

The Medium Energy System (Glycolytic System)

Next up is the glycolytic system, or medium energy system, which is pretty complicated. All you need to know is that this system powers your moderate-to-high intensity, short-duration activities, such as sprinting, lifting weights, playing a sport, or anything else that would feel like a workout. The medium energy system kicks in after about 10 seconds, when the fast energy system runs out, and works for slightly longer—although it still runs out fairly quickly.

ESSENTIAL

Many people believe that sweating during a workout means you are losing fat, which is why people try things like hot yoga to get in shape. If you notice you are several pounds lighter after a workout, odds are that most of that weight was water lost through sweating, not actual fat loss. Always remember to rehydrate yourself and drink plenty of fluids after any activity that causes you to sweat heavily.

This energy system primarily uses glucose produced from stored glycogen. To put it in simpler terms, glucose is a simple sugar molecule, so this system is running on sugar. When you consume carbohydrates, they are stored as glycogen in your muscles. Glycogen is readily available for your body to use during exercise, and while the body can produce it naturally using protein or fat, nothing is faster than having stored glycogen ready to go.

FACT

When you lift weights or strength train, you create an environment where your body will be more inclined to use nutrients for recovery and repair rather than stored fat reserves. Resistance training causes micro damage to your muscles, and your body will be working hard for hours, even days, to repair the damage—a job that burns calories and requires carbs.

Those carbohydrates, in the form of glycogen, are later broken down further into simple sugar molecules that fuel the glycolytic (or medium) energy system. This is why athletes talk about carb-loading before a race or big sporting event; they want to make sure their glycogen stores are filled so their bodies have plenty to draw from.

Even if you aren't an athlete, consuming carbohydrates around your workout is important for maximum performance. Now that you understand how this system works, you should be able to see why. Giving your body readily available fuel in the form of glycogen is essential if you want to run at your highest level.

So what happens if there is no glycogen in the muscles to be used? If you remember, you learned that carbohydrates are not essential for life. If they aren't essential, and you aren't consuming any and storing them as glycogen, how does this medium energy system operate? Well, your body can undergo the complex process of gluconeogenesis. This process involves breaking down stored muscle tissue, ripping it apart, and converting it to glucose. This is a much slower way to get glucose and is not optimal.

FACT

In addition to serving as fuel, carbohydrates play an important role in recovery from training and exercise. After a tough workout, your body switches into recovery mode, as it needs to work hard to repair the damage you did. This repair process requires energy, and giving your body carbs will allow it to do a better job of rebuilding the muscle tissue you broke down.

If you regularly exercise intensely, your best bet is including carbs in your diet, at least on workout days. You *can* work out without carbs, but your performance will suffer, as you won't have that glycogen ready for easy access. Think of your glycogen stores as a fuel tank for the car that is your body and carbohydrates as the fuel. Without fueling up, you'll have a difficult time operating at peak efficiency for any length of time.

The Slow Energy System (Oxidative System)

The last of the big three you need to know about is the oxidative system. This is the slow energy system and provides a sustained release of energy for low-to-moderate activities that last a bit longer. Long runs, swimming, hiking, hot yoga, yard work—these are all activities that are more intense than your resting state but can be sustained for a long time.

This system uses a mixture of carbohydrates and fats for fuel. While carbohydrates are still important and will benefit your body when it's using the oxidative system, they aren't quite as important as they are to the medium energy system.

ESSENTIAL

NEAT, or non-exercise activity thermogenesis, simply refers to the calories burned from any activity that wouldn't be considered traditional exercise. If you hate exercise, there are plenty of ways you can still increase your daily energy output. Park far away from your destination when you go places and walk more, try to stand up periodically throughout the day, and just move more as often as possible.

If you regularly go on long walks, hikes, or swim laps for your exercise, carbs are optional for you. They may help, but your body can also run just fine off of fat during these long-duration exercises. The choice is yours. Carbs are very useful during moderate-to-high intensity, short-duration exercises, but with these easier forms of exercise, carbs aren't quite as important.

The Benefits of the Macronutrient Diet

A flexible diet is adaptable to any lifestyle and schedule. Where most diets are focused solely on fat loss, the macronutrient diet works with any goal, whether that goal is fat loss, muscle gain, athletic performance, or simply general health.

The next section will provide real-life examples of how this diet can be the perfect fit for any lifestyle. It may sound too good to be true; after all, diets aren't supposed to be fun, right?

Well, not only can this diet be fun, but it's also the best option for a sustainable, healthy plan that you could realistically follow for the rest of your life. Most diets are too restrictive and aren't meant to last longer than twelve weeks. If you put in the time to understand and learn how flexible dieting works, you'll know how to eat for optimal health for the rest of your life.

Psychological Benefits

The number one benefit of this diet, and the reason so many people find it sustainable for the long haul, is the lack of restriction. It's not a free-for-all diet and you do need to exercise some self-control and portion control, but you can still eat any food you want, so long as it fits your macro targets for the day.

Freedom to choose what foods you want to eat is a refreshing approach to dieting, and the one that will be the most sustainable. Basic psychology reveals that humans tend to be more drawn to what they aren't supposed to have. If someone walked up and told you that you could never eat your favorite food again, how much more would you crave it? Even if you didn't want it that badly before, knowing it would be off the table forever probably makes you want it.

With flexible dieting this is never an issue. You don't have to have one last cheat day before giving up bread for the summer. You don't have to skip dessert at social events. With the macronutrient diet, if you plan ahead of time and make the correct adjustments, any food you can imagine can fit your plan.

Once you get this diet down, which does take practice and a bit of mental training if you've dieted before, you can start to remove the guilt you may associate with eating "junk" food. It's very common to see someone on a diet slip up and eat something they weren't supposed to, feel guilty and ashamed, and then just blow off the diet completely, promising to start again on Monday. This is a bad cycle and an unnecessary negative association with food. Flexible dieting allows you to break this cycle for good if you take the time to practice it and make it work.

Physical Benefits

From a physical health perspective, flexible dieting is a great way to get in shape and ensure you're getting the proper nutrients you need without any guesswork. The precision required means that if you set up your numbers and food sources properly, you can give your body exactly what it needs to feel and look good day after day.

Other diets tend to take a broad approach; they ask you to eliminate certain food groups, try to control your portions, and hope for the best.

Sometimes this works and sometimes it doesn't, but they don't always ensure you're actually getting the right nutrients.

Simply telling you to cut out processed foods, for example, doesn't mean you'll understand the ins and outs of nutrition and make sure you're eating the right foods every day. Because flexible dieting requires you to get involved and pay attention to what's in all the foods you're eating, you'll learn a lot about nutrition and what's actually in various foods as you begin tracking.

FACT

To avoid getting stuck tracking your macros forever, it's best to automate as much as you can. Find one or two breakfasts you enjoy, one or two lunches you enjoy, and a few snacks. By cycling through these same meals over and over, you'll really only have to worry about measuring and tracking dinner, or whatever your free meal may be.

As far as body composition is concerned, flexible dieting is the most precise way to control your food intake and make small adjustments as needed. If you always have an idea of exactly where your calories are at, as well as your individual macronutrients, it's easy to make a small adjustment, like removing 30 grams of carbs from your daily intake, or adding 10 grams of fat, things like that. An untracked diet makes it impossible to be precise, and this precision is needed to push through plateaus and continue to see results.

Lifestyle Benefits

The number one benefit of the flexible diet is that as long as you track your macros, you can eat any foods you want at any time of the day, and if the numbers add up, you'll still see the changes in your body that you desire. No other diet out there allows this sort of customization to your individual lifestyle.

Time is the biggest reason given for why people can't get in shape. Exercising takes time, cooking healthy meals takes time, and most people have very full schedules. Between work, a social life, and family time, the idea of cooking three to four healthy meals every day and finding time to exercise throughout the week can seem nearly impossible.

FACT

Meal frequency is irrelevant for weight loss. You've probably read over and over that you need to eat four to five small meals spread evenly throughout the day. This simply isn't true. Studies have looked at multiple small meals compared to one or two large meals, and as long as the calories were the same, the results were the same.

With flexible dieting, you can build a meal plan that fits your schedule. If you find you have a very busy morning with no time to eat, you can grab a light snack and save most of your calories for later in the day. If you wake up starving, you can eat a huge breakfast. If you work split shifts or are a student with an irregular schedule, you can simply eat whenever you have a minute to sit down and make the numbers work.

There is no rigid schedule, or strict meal plan to follow. Every part of the macronutrient diet can be tailored to your exact needs and preferences.

How to Indulge and Still See Results

On to the most fun part of the book: how to eat all the foods you love without sabotaging your progress. This may be the only diet in existence that not only allows you to eat your favorite foods but encourages it. You also shouldn't have to use negative words like "cheat meals"; these meals and snacks should fit into your diet without causing you to miss your macros, and as such are perfectly acceptable.

The biggest problem people have is regarding health concerns. You'll hear lots of false claims about artificial sweeteners, processed foods, GMOs, and other "evils" of the food industry. It may be worth addressing those things if you're in the medical field or you have a special condition, but those are irrelevant for most people. Are artificial sweeteners healthy? Probably not. However, their dangers are severely overstated, and unless you're consuming ten cans of diet soda a day, you should be fine. The other fact people tend to overlook is that carrying excess body fat is far more unhealthy than whatever trace ingredients might be in your afternoon snack.

If someone is maintaining a healthy body weight with the occasional vending machine snack or diet soda thrown in, that person is much healthier than the person who's still 40-pounds overweight and worrying about GMOs and artificial sweeteners. This book is meant to help you finally make a lasting change and not get caught up in the minor details. Worry about those little things later.

The truth is, the most effective diet is the one you can stick to for a long time. Making a lasting change takes time, and bouncing from diet to diet, losing and gaining the same five pounds over and over, isn't going to get you anywhere. If having a cookie every night after dinner helps you finally reach your goal weight, that's significantly better than trying to cut out all sweets and resorting to binge eating every weekend, making no long-term progress.

How Much Is Too Much?

Now that you know it's okay to eat fun foods on a regular basis, you need to understand how much of your diet should consist of these treats. The big concern here is overall internal health, not pure weight loss or weight gain.

FACT

If you use a lot of your macros eating foods that are particularly high in carbs and sodium, you may notice the scale jump up seemingly overnight. These foods can cause extra water retention because the high carb and sodium content pulls water into the cells of your body. If you wake up the next day feeling bloated, there's no need to panic. Just drink plenty of water, and your body will balance itself out after a day or two.

If you recall in the section in Chapter 1 about micronutrients, you read that they are vital for internal health. Heart health, bone health, mental health, energy levels, your mood…all of these things and many more rely on adequate nutrition. These micronutrients come from fruits, vegetables, lean meats, healthy fats, and other things that would typically be considered healthy foods.

The issue then with eating processed foods is that they are generally lacking in these micronutrients. Spending your macros on processed foods means you'll have less available for whole foods that provide those good nutrients. Many people try to use a multivitamin or greens supplement as nutritional insurance, which isn't a bad idea, but nothing will be as good as eating whole foods every day.

A good rule is to follow the $^{80}/_{20}$ rule. Eighty percent of the time try to eat whole, unprocessed foods. These are the foods that supply the nutrition you need to feel your best. The other 20 percent of the time, have some fun. Think of a few treats you love and figure out how to work them into your meal plan. You can do a small treat every day, or eat whole foods most of the week and have one or two fun meals. The choice is yours. Just keep in mind that the more processed foods you eat, the greater risk you have of feeling less that optimal, as you're lowering your nutrient intake.

CHAPTER 4

Macronutrients for Better Health

The previous three chapters have explained how macronutrients function. Now that you have a big-picture understanding of how nutrition works, it's time to look at how to eat for maximum health. While calories are the biggest factor in weight loss or weight gain, if you're concerned with your overall well-being, understanding the details of how these foods affect your body is very important.

Choose Whole Foods over Processed Foods

The biggest selling point of the macronutrient diet is that this style of flexible dieting allows you to enjoy the foods you love, guilt-free. Well, as long as you account for them and make sure you don't overeat.

It's been clearly shown that total energy balance, or calories in versus calories out, is what determines weight loss. There are no evil foods or special rules about how many meals you need to eat. Food you eat after six p.m. isn't automatically going to make you fat, and plenty of people have lost significant weight using a diet composed of mostly fast foods or processed snacks.

Just because this works does not mean it's ideal. Sure, you can lose fat, but if you want your body to run at 100 percent efficiency and be healthy on the inside as well, it's important to make sure you're getting the right foods in your diet. Flexible dieting doesn't mean that you *have* to eat the fun foods and snacks; it just means that you *can*.

If you understand that calories are what matter, you may not understand all the reasons why whole-food sources are more beneficial than packaged, processed foods. Before looking at the details of each macronutrient, you need to know why whole foods are important to include in your diet when it comes to helping you stay on track and make the right choices.

Synergistic Nutrition

The most important reason for choosing whole foods is the micronutrients they contain. Micronutrients are the vitamins and minerals that support all of your body's important functions, like muscular contractions, mental functioning, and a healthy immune system. Without proper micronutrients, you may look fine on the outside, but you're not giving your body everything it needs to be healthy on the inside.

Vitamins and minerals can be obtained through pills and powders, but nothing works as well as getting them from your food. Many minerals work together to enhance each other, and whole foods often contain the vitamins and minerals that work well together.

As an example, vitamin D is often found in fatty food sources as it requires fat intake to be absorbed. If you try to supplement with vitamin D, you have to make sure you take it with a fatty meal, something nature takes care of for you with whole foods. This holds true for all kinds of vitamins and minerals that your body needs to function.

Whole Foods Are More Filling

Eating whole, unprocessed food groups, like fruits, vegetables, and lean meats, are an excellent way to stay full when dieting. One of the biggest concerns with losing fat is hunger. When you find yourself running low on calories but still very hungry, it's important to make sure the calories you're consuming will keep you feeling full. Walking around hungry will only make it that much harder to say no to foods that aren't part of your plan.

Fruits and vegetables often contain significant amounts of fiber. This fiber slows down the digestion process, helping you feel full and satisfied hours after you eat. With whole-food protein sources like meat and eggs, your body has to work very hard to break down the food. This is why a steak fills you up a lot more than a bowl of pasta.

FACT

The one time a supplement would be useful instead of a whole food or as an addition to your diet is when you're using protein powder. Protein powders are made from foods, like dairy and egg products, and they contain enough macros and calories to be considered a food source in their own right. These powders shouldn't replace your whole-food protein intake, but if you're struggling to hit your protein numbers, a supplement can be a useful tool.

Nutritional Accuracy

Lastly, nutritional accuracy is very important when tracking macronutrients. If you plan to eat a variety of foods, throw in some treats from time to time, and still come close to your macro goals every day, you'd better know exactly what you're eating.

Nutritional labels are usually close but are not 100 percent accurate, and there's no way to really know what you're getting. You're probably fine if you're eating foods out of packages, but then you're also getting a whole lot of other added, unnecessary ingredients.

The accuracy concern is particularly true with restaurants or fast food chains. Many chain restaurants have nutritional information available online, which is a good guess but usually not accurate. Depending on the chef, a meal may have different nutritional values every time you eat it, so even if you track that meal, it's just an educated guess.

Whenever possible, prepare your own meals using whole-food ingredients. Even if your measurements aren't perfect, you'll still be in a much better place than simply hoping the restaurant calculations are accurate or existing solely off of packaged snack foods.

What about the glycemic index?
There is a lot of misinformation in the mainstream media about the glycemic index of carbs, with many claiming that high-glycemic carbs are bad and low-glycemic carbs are good. In reality, the glycemic index simply measures how fast carbs digest, which is a process slowed by fiber. High-fiber carbs will generally be lower on the glycemic index and keep you feeling full longer; however, fast-digesting carbs are not all bad and shouldn't be feared.

Fiber-Rich Carbohydrates

When it comes to carbohydrates, the biggest concern is fiber content. High-fiber carbs, like oats, whole grains, and green vegetables, are excellent for your digestive system and keeping you full. Adequate fiber intake is also associated with improved heart health and blood sugar levels.

There are two kinds of fiber, soluble fiber and insoluble fiber. Insoluble fiber is a tough, dense fiber that can't be broken down by the gut. It moves through the digestive system, adding bulk to your waste, which promotes regular bowel movements. This fiber is commonly found in dense leafy greens, the skin of fruits and vegetables, and certain whole grains.

Soluble fiber absorbs water and liquid and has many benefits when consumed in the proper quantity. As it absorbs water, it forms a thick, gel-like substance. In addition to this gel helping keep you regular and feeling full, soluble fiber can bind to sugar and cholesterol, slowing or completely preventing their absorption into the bloodstream. This is why high-fiber diets can lower blood sugar and cholesterol levels, which in turn reduces the risk of heart disease later in life.

ALERT

Because soluble fiber absorbs water, it's very important to consume plenty of liquids when eating fibrous foods. Any time you eat a high-fiber meal, like a large salad or a bowl of oatmeal, make sure you drink an extra glass of water or two. If too much fiber is consumed, it can absorb too much liquid from your digestive system, causing cramping, an upset stomach, and constipation. Eat your fiber but take care to stay hydrated.

Ideally, fiber should come from the foods you eat. You can supplement with fiber, but this can commonly cause digestive issues and stomach cramping. Most adults should aim for 20–30 grams of fiber in their diet each day, a very obtainable number with the right foods. If you're reaching this number through your regular diet, there's no need to supplement with fiber, and taking more could simply end up irritating your digestive system.

Lean Proteins

Of all the nutrients, protein may be the most misunderstood. People are quick to vilify carbohydrates and fats, claiming they are all sorts of evil, but no one seems to know what to think about protein. Some say it damages your liver; others say you need incredibly high amounts of protein in your diet.

The answer is somewhere in the middle. Protein in proper quantities won't have any negative effects, but you probably don't need as much as most people claim. For optimal recovery from training, satiety, and a healthy body, 1 gram of protein per pound of lean body weight is a pretty good guideline.

Your lean body mass is your total body weight minus body fat. It's very hard to calculate this number perfectly without advanced testing, but you can try. Figure out your body fat percentage from measuring using a handheld device, a digital scale that tracks body fat, or get a local trainer at your gym to measure your body fat. If none of these are options, you can search online for body fat measurement pictures. Your total body weight times your body fat percentage will tell you how many pounds of fat you carry, and your total weight minus fat calculation gives you your lean body mass weight.

At a minimum, .6 grams of protein will keep you feeling okay. Fewer than that, and you may start to experience negative side effects. Not getting enough protein can cause you to lose muscle, as your body will break down your muscle tissue for the amino acids it contains.

The rest of this section will look at some of the most popular and readily available protein sources and go into a little bit of detail about each. It's important to know the basics of protein sources so that you can be sure to choose the most optimal ones for your health and well-being.

Guide to Meat Sources

The most common source of protein is going to be meat. These are your chicken, turkey, pork, and beef meals. Meats are going to be complete sources of protein, which means they contain all of the essential amino acids your body needs that must be obtained from foods.

Poultry

With poultry like chicken and turkey, the quality isn't quite as important as their fat content. Whenever possible, go for the cuts with the least amount of fat possible. Lean ground turkey, lean turkey breast, and boneless, skinless chicken breasts are all great options.

Both chicken and turkey can be prepared with virtually zero added fat, which can be a nice alternative to beef products, which have fat that is much harder to remove. While the skin can be quite fatty, it's okay to enjoy it as long as you account for the fat. It's also very easy to cook chicken with the skin to retain the meat's moisture and flavor, and then just remove it before eating.

Should I be looking for cage-free and organic chicken products?
With chicken, this isn't very important in terms of nutritional benefit. Unfortunately, chicken labeled cage-free simply means it needs to have unlimited access to food and water and minimal space to roam during the laying cycle, not that it actually lives outside of its cage and eats real food. Also, most of the toxins in your chicken are stored in the fat, which is easy to trim and remove, so even lower-cost chicken can be quite healthy if properly prepared. The exception is eggs; cage-free eggs with dark yolks will have more nutrition than mass-produced, lightly colored eggs. The darker yolk comes from the higher quantities of micronutrients, so if you encounter an egg with a dark yolk, don't be alarmed.

Pork
When it comes to pork, try to stick to lean pork chops or pork loin. Other sources of pork like bacon or sausages are fine to eat, but they'll generally have high fat to protein ratios, which can make it a bit harder to fit into your daily macros. Many people tend to vilify pork, but if you choose a lean cut and prepare it correctly, it's perfectly fine to enjoy.

Beef
Whenever possible, choose grass-fed beef sources. This costs a bit more, but the nutritional benefit is much better, and the flavor tends to be a bit richer and more powerful. There are several reasons why grass-fed beef is beneficial, and if you can make room for it in your budget, it's significantly better than farm-raised beef.

Cows raised on farms are generally kept in small pens and fed grain-heavy diets, which can lead to beef that is lacking in nutrients. Cows that are free to graze on grass and move around a bit more will have more nutrients from all the greens and tend to provide leaner and healthier cuts of beef, as the cows get more exercise and fresh air. Grass-fed beef is high in omega-3 fatty acids, which are anti-inflammatory, as well as CLA, or conjugated linoleic acid, a fatty acid associated with healthy body fat levels.

Healthy Fats

By now you should understand that fat is not evil; rather, it's a necessary component of a diet for optimal long-term health. The right sources of fat keep your hormones functioning, your brain operating on all cylinders, your skin healthy, and your joints and cells protected. Fat is important.

Not all fat is good, however. While you should be adding fat to your diet, it's vital to make sure you're getting the right fats in the right balances. This section will take a closer look at the various types of fat, where they come from, and how to properly balance them.

As a refresher, it's important to understand the benefits of healthy fats, just to make sure you aren't still scared of enjoying them.

BENEFITS OF HEALTHY FATS
- Improved reproductive health
- Improved hormone production
- Improved brain function
- Decreased inflammation
- Improved skin health
- Improved cellular health
- Improved cholesterol levels

Yes, fat may contain the most calories, but without dietary fat, your body would slowly begin to shut down. You don't need too much, but you definitely need to make sure you're getting at least some forms of fat in your diet on a regular basis.

ESSENTIAL

Saturated fats are not bad fats, at least not in the proper amounts, but they aren't exactly good, either. Saturated fats are typically found in red meat, as well as in certain dairy products. You do need some saturated fats, and it would be pretty hard to avoid them completely, but try to limit them. They won't kill you, like some claim, but they aren't as good as the unsaturated fats.

Saturated, Unsaturated, or Something Else?

Fat gets confusing, and for good reason—there are quite a few types. You don't really need to understand how exactly these are classified; you just need to understand the difference between good and bad fats.

To start, trans fat is the only truly bad fat. Trans fats are found in fried and processed foods and usually have negative effects on your cholesterol and heart health. Whenever possible, avoid any food containing trans fats. Most trans fats are artificially created, so if you see that a food contains trans fats, put it down and walk away.

When it comes to good fats, unsaturated fats are the ones you want. You'll see monounsaturated and polyunsaturated fats, and these are both good types of fat. Unsaturated fats have been shown to lower levels of bad cholesterol while promoting levels of good cholesterol. If you're trying to eat the fats generally classified as healthy, like whole eggs, nuts, and avocados, you should be getting plenty of unsaturated fats.

Lastly, you should make every possible effort to get as many omega-3 fatty acids as you can. These are very anti-inflammatory; good for your heart, skin, and brain; and will help you achieve a better quality of life. You can get your omega-3s from high-quality fish oil supplements or just by making an effort to eat wild-caught fish two to three times per week.

Micronutrient Balance

Micronutrients, as you learned, are the many vitamins and minerals found in foods. They give you energy, support your body at a cellular level, boost your immune system, fight aging, and are very important for feeling and looking your best.

However, just because you eat a few fruits and vegetables doesn't necessarily mean you're covered. There are a lot of vitamins and minerals out there, and you need to make sure you're getting all of the essentials. If you become deficient in any micronutrients, you might not notice a difference right away, but you'll probably notice side effects over time—effects that can get quite serious.

While you could supplement with a multivitamin or greens powder, you'll get much more value from eating a variety of whole foods to get your micronutrients. Supplements are made to supplement a healthy diet, not replace any part of it, so while they aren't bad, you shouldn't use supplements as an excuse to not eat your fruits and vegetables.

ALERT

Just because you eat a lot of vegetables doesn't mean you're getting enough micronutrients. It's the quality that matters, not the quantity. Eating chicken and broccoli three times a day may keep you well within your macronutrient targets, but you're only getting the nutrients from broccoli in that example. Don't fall into the bad habit of only eating a few vegetables; make an effort to eat as many as possible.

To help you get your nutrients in, here are a few strategies that can help you stay on track with your goals and ensure you're getting the right variety. Your diet may never be perfect, but you can always work to make it as healthy as possible. These strategies will help you.

Eat the Rainbow

This isn't referring to a popular candy; it refers to eating all the colored fruits and vegetables you can get your hands on. Fruits and vegetables often get their color from micronutrients. For example, foods high in beta-carotene often appear orange, like carrots and sweet potatoes.

This sounds complicated to do, but it's easier than it seems. Keeping mixed bell peppers on hand, either fresh or frozen for stir-fries, is an easy way to get your red, green, yellow, and orange vegetables in. Combine this with some mixed berries for antioxidants with a few meals and plenty of leafy greens, like spinach, kale, and broccoli, and you'll be well on your way to a nutritious diet.

Eat Fruits or Vegetables at Every Meal

If you find it hard to get enough fruits and vegetables in your diet, make it a habit to eat a serving of fruits or vegetables with every main meal. Oftentimes people will eat a salad or vegetables with dinner but opt for quick and easy meals for breakfast and lunch. This is fine, but there's always a way to add more nutritional value to your meals.

With breakfast, the easiest way to do this is by keeping fruit on hand. Oranges, apples, bananas, kiwis, berries, and pears are all very healthy fruits that are absolutely packed with nutrients. These fruits are easy to eat and can also be carried around for a quick and healthy snack throughout the day.

For lunch and dinner, salads and vegetables are your friend. It's very easy to throw several handfuls of mixed greens and spinach into a bowl, top with some low-fat dressing, and enjoy. Not only will this provide a large dose of antioxidants and nutrients, but it will keep you feeling full between meals.

If you really struggle with this, a multivitamin or greens powder may be helpful, but those should never be your main source of nutrition, just a backup insurance policy. Make an effort to get your micronutrients in every single day, and your body will thank you.

CHAPTER 5

How to Build Your Perfect Diet

In order to build your perfect diet plan, you must first decide what your goals are. Are you looking to just lose weight? Are you looking to gain more muscle? Your final goal will influence your eating plan and how many macros you will require each day. Once you have your goals in mind, this chapter will show you how to calculate the proper amount of calories and macronutrients that you should be eating each day. With your macronutrient amounts calculated, you can then create your eating plan, including what times you should eat and what your meals should consist of. Proper planning is key to success on the macronutrient diet, so let's get started.

Weight Loss versus Muscle Gain Macronutrient Formulas

Whether your goal is to lose weight or build some muscle, you'll need to adjust your current calorie intake. Remember that losing fat requires a caloric deficit, or eating less than you burn in a day. The opposite is true for building muscle—you need to eat more than you need and give your body the extra food it needs to grow.

In general, you can be a bit more aggressive when trying to lose fat than when trying to gain muscle. While it is possible to lose weight too quickly, it's much more preferable to lose weight fast and adjust to slow it down. You'll just look better faster.

FACT

Body composition simply refers to the ratio of fat to lean tissue you carry. A higher body fat percentage means that more of your total body weight comes from fat, as opposed to lean tissue, bones, and organs. When someone mentions improving body composition, they are generally referring to reducing body fat while maintaining, or even building, lean muscle tissue. Improving body composition is the fastest way to visually look better and get other people noticing that your body is changing.

With muscle building, you should take a slow, controlled approach. Start with only small increases, see how your body responds, and increase again as needed. A common mistake is for people to start eating everything in sight when they want to build muscle and then end up gaining more body fat than they intended. When building muscle, the goal is to build actual muscle—not simply make the scale move up by gaining fat as well.

Eating for Performance

As you assemble your meal plan, consider your primary goal. Is it body composition and the number on the scale or performing your best during your workouts or athletic activities?

For pure body composition, meal timing doesn't matter at all. As long as your numbers add up at the end of the day, you'll be just fine. If you are trying to lose weight without exercising and focus only on your nutrition, you can set up your meal plan however you'd like without worrying about meal timing.

If you're an active person and want to perform your best and recover from your exercise, meal timing comes into play a bit more. As discussed in Chapter 3, carbohydrates play a large role in both fueling your exercise and helping you recover. It makes sense then to place a significant portion of your carbohydrates before and after intense physical activity, as this will give you the most benefit from them. This is especially important if you're dieting, and your carbohydrates are getting lower and lower.

For high-intensity activities such as working out, running, or playing a sport, use carbs to fuel your workouts for maximum benefit. You should try to consume at least 30–40 percent of them an hour before your workout and 30–40 percent immediately after. Any remaining carbohydrates can be spread around the day however you prefer.

How to Find Your Exact Numbers

It's time to get into the actual numbers. You'll start by figuring out your maintenance calorie intake, which is roughly how many calories your body uses every day. To lose fat, you'll eat fewer calories than your maintenance levels, and to build muscle, you'll eat above maintenance.

QUESTION

Why do women need fewer calories than men?
Women naturally have lower levels of muscle than men do. They don't have quite as much testosterone and growth hormone, either, so building muscle is a bit more challenging. Because muscle tissue burns calories even at rest, the higher levels of muscle in men, along with higher levels of testosterone and growth hormone, mean that men typically burn more calories per pound than women do.

There are many ways to do this, and none will ever be 100 percent accurate. So, to figure out your fat loss calories, which you'll need to track and adjust as you go, you'll need a bit of trial and error in the beginning. Keep in mind that so many factors affect your caloric output—activity levels, genetics, body composition, nutrition, and many more. The math you're about to do will be a best guess, so don't expect to get your calories perfect on the first try. There will also be a walk-through at the end of this section using a fictional character, so you can follow along with your own numbers.

Step One: Figure Out Your Total Calories

There are plenty of complicated, long calculations out there, but you can keep it simple. If you're a man, multiply your body weight by 14. If you're a woman, multiply your body weight by 12. This will give you a rough guess at your total calories needed to maintain your body weight.

Now that you've come up with a number for your calories, the next step is to consume calories according to this number as closely as you can for seven to ten days. Check your body weight on day one and day ten to compare.

If you lose weight, you've found a caloric deficit. If fat loss is your goal, this is perfect. If you lost more than two and a half pounds, however, that's too fast, and you're undereating. You'll want to bump food up a bit.

If you gained weight, you're eating above maintenance. Lower your food intake by a few hundred calories and try again. You want to start with a 15 percent decrease in calories, eat that number for a few days, and then check your weight again, repeating until you find your maintenance level.

If your weight stayed the same, you found your maintenance intake. To lose fat, take about 500 calories away from your total carbs and fats. If you want to add muscle, add about 300 calories primarily to carbs with some going to fat.

Step Two: Calculate Your Macros

Now that you have your total calories, it's time to split those calories up into their respective macros. Remember, protein and carbohydrates each have four calories per gram, while fat has nine calories per gram. If you want to plan to include alcohol, it has seven calories per gram but zero nutritional value, so you'll have to lower your remaining calories and simply eat less carbs and fat.

- **Protein:** Set your protein at 1 gram per pound of lean body weight. Write that number down.
- **Fat:** Now set your fat anywhere between .25–.45 grams per pound (lower if you prefer higher carbs, and vice versa).
- **Carbs:** Your remaining calories, after protein and fat, will go to carbs. On training days, set your carbs at 1.25–1.5 grams per pound of body weight, depending on how you ended up setting your fat (higher or lower). On rest days, set your carbs at .5 grams per pound and increase fat by .10 grams per pound.

While protein should stay the same, your fat and carbs can fluctuate based on your personal preference. If you enjoy fatty foods, keep your fat at .45 grams per pound or even higher. This will lower your carbohydrate intake but give you room for foods you enjoy. If you love carbs, keep your fat on the lowest end, .25 grams per pound, and you can enjoy pasta to your heart's content.

Macro Calculation Example

Let's take a 200-pound male with a measured 15 percent body fat and calculate his macros using the previous numbers. Reading the process can seem overwhelming, but following an example will show you how simple it really is.

First and foremost, let's calculate lean body mass. This will be used to determine protein intake. The reason you calculate for lean mass rather than total body weight is to feed your body based on its needs. Since body fat is not active tissue, it doesn't need any nutrition to sustain itself. The rest of your lean mass, consisting of your muscular system, internal organs, bones, and anything that's not fat, does in fact need proper nutrition to function, so that's what you should be concerned with regarding your protein needs.

Total Calorie Calculations

For total calories, use 14 times total body weight for men, so for the sample calculations, total maintenance calories will be 2,800.

For fat loss, it's best to start with a 500-calorie per day deficit. Therefore, our fictional man's total calorie intake goals will be 2,300 calories per day.

For the rest of the calculations, use the following conversion chart.

MACRO TO CALORIE CONVERSIONS

- 1 gram protein = 4 calories
- 1 gram carbohydrate = 4 calories
- 1 gram fat = 9 calories

Lean Body Mass Calculation

1. Total body weight × body fat percentage = pounds of fat
2. Total body weight – pounds of fat = lean body mass

Remember, the sample person weighs 200 pounds at 15 percent body fat.

1. 200 × .15 (15 percent) = 30 pounds of fat
2. 200 pounds – 30 pounds = 170 pounds lean body mass

Protein Calculations

Protein should be set at 1 gram per pound of lean body weight. At 170 pounds of lean body mass, this means protein will be set at 170 grams every day.

Protein calories are 170 × 4, or 680.

Fat Calculations

Fat should be set at .25–.45 grams per pound of body weight. Since the man weighs 200 pounds and prefers higher-fat meals, he'll use .45 grams: 200 pounds × .45 grams means fat will be set at 90 grams per day.

Fat calories are 90 × 9, or 810.

Carbohydrate Calculations

To calculate carbohydrates, take your protein and fat calories and subtract them from your total calories for the day. The remaining calories are used for carbohydrates.

Total calories – protein calories – fat calories = carbohydrate calories.

2,300 – 680 – 810 = 810 carbohydrate calories.

Now that you have 810 carbohydrate calories, simply divide this number by 4 to figure out how many grams of carbohydrates are to be consumed each day:

810 ÷ 4 = 203 grams of carbohydrates every day.

Therefore, the final goal numbers for each day are 2,300 calories, coming from 170 grams of protein, 90 grams of fat, and 203 grams of carbohydrates.

Use these calculations to figure out your individual daily needs for total calories and total macros and use those numbers to plan your days and meal plans.

Remember, these numbers are just a best guess and will have to be adjusted as you go. Once you get in the habit of accurately consuming these numbers, which takes practice, it's very easy to adjust your diet when progress stalls. Our fictional man could simply go from eating 203 carbs each day to eating 170 carbs each day, for example. Rather than overhauling your entire diet every few weeks and trying something new, you can simply adjust your ratios whenever progress stops.

Build Your Perfect Meal Plan

There's a famous quote about planning that states:

Failing to plan is planning to fail.

When it comes to dietary adherence, this is 100 percent true. If you aren't planning your nutrition ahead of time, there's no way you can have any shot at consistently hitting your macros. Rather than take a reactive approach to your diet and adjust as you go, be proactive and plan your days ahead of time. This way, before the day even starts, you'll see exactly what your macro intake will look like, and you can plan ahead to fill any gaps, or adjust as needed.

If you prefer a more rigid schedule, try planning out two or three perfect days that hit your macros dead-on, and then just follow those meal plans. When coming up with your plans, make sure at least 80 percent of your food is unprocessed, whole foods and make sure it's realistic.

If you work the night shift at a hospital, your food choices and meal frequency will be different than someone who works from home and has access to a kitchen; there really is no one-size-fits-all approach. Plan ahead, make this process as painless and thought-free as possible, and you'll be good to go.

ESSENTIAL

Remember that it's okay to enjoy life, and you shouldn't feel guilty, especially if you plan ahead. If you start to feel guilty, it's easy to bring yourself down, and the temptation to just give up entirely is much stronger. Plan ahead, do your best, and if you slip up, just get back on track as soon as you can.

There are sample meal plans at the end of this book, but if you want to start from scratch, here are the basic steps.

Step One: Figure Out Your Schedule

Start by looking at an average day in your life. How many meals can you eat? When are you the busiest? When do you have the most time to cook?

If you work from home, chances are you'll have an easier time preparing three to four meals per day. If you're a busy executive who's constantly working long days and rushing in and out of meetings, you may find that you need a quick and easy breakfast, a few snacks, and a big dinner.

Regardless of your schedule, figure out what sort of meal plan would be easy for you to follow in terms of timing and write those meals down, times and all.

Step Two: Divide Your Macros

Now that you have your meal times, and total number of meals, attempt to evenly split your macros across each meal. If your goal is 140 grams of protein per day, and you eat four meals, you'd want to aim for around 35 grams with each meal. This makes hitting your macros much more manageable, rather than trying to get all of your protein at once.

If you're working out that day, put most of your carbs before and after your workout, otherwise you can spread them around however you'd like. For each meal, write down the total number of macronutrients and calories you'll need for that meal.

Step Three: Choose Your Foods

Finally, you have the framework. Time to fill it in. Look at each meal and figure out what foods will give you that meal's required calories and macros. This is where you can have fun and get really creative.

The recipes in this book include nutrition calculations that will tell you exactly how many macros are in each serving. This makes planning easy, though of course you can use any food you like.

If you don't want to follow premade recipes, a simple trick is to pick three carbs, three proteins, and two to three high-fat foods to keep around your house at all times. This way, you can mix and match ingredients to plan your meals as needed. Most foods will have the nutritional information right on the package. For produce, nearly all fruits are higher in carbohydrates, while green vegetables will have fewer carbohydrates. For your carbs, you can choose fruit, rice, oats, and potatoes, for example, with your proteins coming from meats, eggs, and maybe protein powder. You can choose different combinations of foods, adding fat as needed through things like cooking oils and butter, or choosing higher-fat cuts of meat, like red meat or fatty fish.

ESSENTIAL

When choosing food sources, keep in mind that foods high in fiber will keep you full the longest, making it easier to diet. Choose leafy greens, whole grains, and assorted fruits and vegetables to fight off hunger during the day.

If you're making a recipe or meal that doesn't have the calculated macros, simply add up all the ingrdients you're using, divide by the number of servings the meal provides, and use those numbers as your macronutrient intake for the meal.

By the end of all this planning, you should have a sample meal plan that fits your schedule perfectly, allows you hit your macros, and uses foods of your choosing—not random foods from a magazine meal plan. You can write out the foods you want by hand, or use an app for a food log, like MyFitnessPal or My Macros+. This way you can plan the next day ahead of time and see where any gaps may be that you need to fill. Planning, and sticking to the plan, sets you up for the best possible chance at success as it's a plan perfectly engineered for your needs, schedule, and preferences.

Adjusting Your Numbers for Continuing Progress

The road to your dream body won't be without its share of ups and downs. It's very normal for your progress to stall, and this should be expected. The human body is incredibly smart and has adapted to survive extreme situations.

While something like trying to lose a bit of belly fat may not seem like the end of the world, your body simply sees a diet as a period of restricted food, and it will act accordingly. Typically, a few weeks of reduced food intake will trigger your body to learn to function at its new calorie level and any weight loss will slow down.

QUESTION

If I diet too long, will I damage my metabolism?
While it's true that your body's metabolism will slow down the longer you diet, it's not necessarily true metabolic damage. After all, both your body weight and food intake will be lowered, so it makes sense that your metabolism will slow down. Unless you have a history of eating disorders or have dieted down to dangerously low levels multiple times, you probably don't have real metabolic damage—you just need to lower your calories.

This could be due to several reasons. Most likely, your body's metabolism has simply adjusted, and because you now weigh less, you don't need

70

as much food, so weight loss will slow down. In more extreme cases of prolonged, severe caloric restriction, it's possible that your body will actually fight weight loss because it thinks that it's not getting enough food, so it wants to hang on to the energy stores it has.

Regardless of the reason, when these situations pop up, it's important to understand how to adjust your diet so that you can continue to make progress toward your goal. If you want to increase that energy deficit so you continue to burn fat, you can either reduce your food intake or work to burn more calories. If you have the time to add some extra cardio sessions to your weekly schedule, that's fine, but it's important to know how to adjust your diet.

When to Adjust

For both weight loss and weight gain, it's rarely a linear process. Over the course of a week, it's very common for your body weight to fluctuate on a daily basis. Hormonal issues, sodium intake, hydration levels, food that's still being processed through your digestion and waste system…all of these factors can increase or decrease the number you see on your scale.

It's best to weigh yourself only once per week at the most. Pick a day and time that you know will be consistent. Some people prefer Monday weigh-ins, although you may be a bit heavier if you ate foods over the weekend that aren't normally part of your diet. Others prefer midweek or Friday weigh-ins, as this lets your body settle into a normal routine, allowing for a more accurate reading.

FACT

If you feel the need to weigh yourself every day, be sure that you won't be upset by daily weight fluctuations. The number on the scale doesn't reflect the whole picture and is just one tool for progress tracking. If you can objectively weigh yourself daily with no negative thoughts, then look at weekly averages. From Monday to Monday your weight might go up and down, but if your average weight is decreasing week after week, you're on the right track.

Regardless of how often you weigh yourself, dietary changes should only be implemented when your weight has plateaued for ten to fourteen days at a minimum. Don't assume that simply because you gained a pound seemingly overnight that you need to immediately lower your calories. Look at the overall trend of your body's weight and only adjust once it's stopped trending in the right direction for about two weeks.

How to Adjust

Start by adjusting your carbohydrates first. As these are the only nonessential macronutrient, most adjustments should come from carbohydrates. Whether your goal is fat loss or muscle gain, the simplest method is to set protein and fat at optimal levels for health and performance and then simply manipulate your carbohydrate intake up or down, based on your goal.

Start with a 10 percent total calorie adjustment. If you've been dieting at 2,000 calories and you've been stuck for two weeks, adjust your calories down to 1,800. This may not be aggressive enough, but it's always better to go slowly and take your time rather than slash your food intake too low, too quickly.

Remember, a gram of carbohydrate has 4 calories. With some simple math you can figure out how many carbs you need to remove. From the previous example, a 200-calorie decrease would mean taking away 50 carbs from the diet.

If your carbs are already very low, you can take calories from protein and fat, but this should be avoided. At a bare minimum, you should be aiming for about .6 grams of protein per pound of body weight, and .2 grams of fat per pound. Ideally those numbers would be a bit higher, but as long as you never dip below those minimums, you should feel okay.

If you reach the point where your proteins and fats are at their minimum, and your carbohydrate intake is already very low, you may need to start adding more exercise. This situation is rare and is usually only seen when people attempt to take their bodies from lean and healthy to very lean with dangerously low levels of body fat, but it can occur. Most people will be able to reach their goal weight without such drastic measures, assuming there are no other major health issues.

Macronutrients and Exercise

The biggest factor that affects the macronutrient ratio you choose is exercise. While exercise is not necessary for weight loss, it's very beneficial and will make the process significantly easier. Exercise is important for overall health and longevity as it improves many health markers beyond the number on the scale.

Here's the thing: exercise uses energy. Physically intense activities, like going for a run or taking a boot camp class, are going to put a much higher energy demand on your body compared to sitting at a desk or laying in bed. As such, it's important to adequately fuel your body.

As discussed earlier, carbohydrates are the best fuel source for exercise. High-intensity activities are fueled primarily by glucose, stored in the body as glycogen. Providing the body with adequate glucose by eating enough carbs is much more efficient than waiting for your body to convert fat and protein to glucose.

Fast-digesting carbohydrates give you both the fuel you need to perform and the materials you need to recover and rebuild. Placing carbohydrates before and after your workouts is the easiest way to make sure you can work hard and recover as fast as possible.

ESSENTIAL

When it comes to workouts, simple carbohydrates are best. Fruits, rice, bread, or sports drinks are excellent options. Avoid foods that contain too much fiber or fat, as both of these can slow down digestion, because your priority is digesting those carbs so that your body can use them. While high-fiber carbs like oatmeal or leafy vegetables are fine, they may not be optimal for immediately before and after workouts.

When planning your meals, be sure to put carbs before and after workouts on your exercise days. Aim for at least 30–50 grams of carbohydrates before and after. If your total carbs are getting low, try to keep as many as you can centered around that workout, as that's when you'll be the most efficient at using them.

How to Enjoy Foods You Love, Guilt-Free

Time to learn how to eat any food you can think of and still make progress. The beauty of the macronutrient diet lies in the freedom to choose what you enjoy, but it must be done correctly. The biggest mistake you can make is seeing a food you love, eating as much of it as you want, and then trying to clean up the mess later (i.e., planning the rest of the day around your indulgence).

Not only can an unplanned indulgence send you way over your daily or even weekly calories, but this is the most common cause of dietary guilt. If you've been tracking your macros consistently and suddenly you get thrown way off track by a cheat meal, it can make you feel like a failure, and it'll be hard to get back on track. This is dangerous for long-term success.

The trick to eating foods you enjoy is planning ahead. If you know that tomorrow night is pizza night, open up tomorrow's food log, plug in however much pizza you want to eat, and adjust the rest of your day accordingly. Being proactive about this will allow you to go through your day stress-free, knowing you'll hit your targets even with that added pizza, and you can enjoy your treat without feeling bad.

QUESTION

What about vacations? Should I track my food and stick to the plan on vacation?
This is a completely personal decision. If you loosely track your food and try to control your portions throughout the day, you can certainly have fun while minimizing the "damage" and avoid coming home ten pounds heavier. However, if you prefer to indulge in whatever you want on your trip, know that this is completely fine. It just may take a bit of time when you return home to get things back on track.

This works for anything, not just pizza. Plan it ahead of time and adjust your day to fit that treat in. It takes moderation, but it can be done. Once you get comfortable with planning small treats and indulgences into your diet, you'll soon realize that the macronutrient diet doesn't require you to give up any of your favorite foods or drinks; you just have to make room for them.

CHAPTER 6

Breakfast and Brunch

Low-Carb Protein Waffle

This tasty breakfast will satisfy your cravings without giving you any unnecessary carbohydrates. Choose a protein flavor you like, as this will influence the final flavor.

INGREDIENTS | SERVES 1

1 scoop whey protein (any flavor)
1 teaspoon baking powder
1 teaspoon cinnamon
1 large egg
½ cup water

Top It with Flavor

This waffle is very low calorie and can be topped with butter, whipped cream, syrup, fresh fruit, or any other topping you love. If you have higher carbs on waffle day, top it with fresh fruit and maybe some natural maple syrup. If it's a low-carb day, you can top it with some nut butters or whipped cream to add some flavor and nutrition.

1. Preheat a waffle maker for 5 minutes.

2. Add whey protein, baking powder, and cinnamon to a medium bowl and mix well.

3. Add egg and mix well with a fork.

4. Add water and mix well; more can be added to reach your desired consistency.

5. Cook 45–60 seconds in the waffle maker and serve immediately.

Per Serving | Calories: 185 | Fat: 5 g | Protein: 31 g | Sodium: 602 mg | Fiber: 1.5 g | Carbohydrates: 5 g | Sugar: 1 g

Peaches and Cream Oatmeal

This spin on a classic dish is a refreshing breakfast for those hot summer mornings, and it packs a protein punch.

INGREDIENTS | SERVES 1

1¼ cups water
½ cup dry quick-cooking oats
1 scoop vanilla whey protein
½ cup skim milk
1 packet stevia
1 medium peach, peeled, pitted, and sliced

The Power of Oatmeal

Oatmeal is very high in fiber, so it will keep you feeling full all morning long while providing a slow, sustained release of energy. Because of its fiber content, oatmeal can absorb a lot of water, so be sure to stay hydrated and drink 1–2 big glasses of water with each serving. If you find you have digestive issues with oats, you can try switching to Cream of Wheat or Cream of Rice for a warm breakfast alternative.

1. Combine water and oats in a medium microwave-safe bowl.

2. Cook in microwave on high 3 minutes or until desired texture is reached.

3. In a separate bowl or shaker cup, mix protein and milk, then add to the cooked oats and stir. Add stevia and mix well.

4. Top with peaches and serve immediately.

Per Serving | Calories: 368 | Fat: 4.5 g | Protein: 36 g | Sodium: 105 mg | Fiber: 6 g | Carbohydrates: 51 g | Sugar: 20 g

Apple Oatmeal Pancakes

Pancakes are a fun treat that can be prepared in a wide variety of ways.
This recipe has added protein and fruit to keep you full and energized.

INGREDIENTS | MAKES 4 PANCAKES

6 large egg whites
½ cup oatmeal
1 tablespoon unsweetened applesauce
1 teaspoon cinnamon
1 packet stevia
¼ teaspoon baking soda
1 teaspoon olive oil
1 medium apple, diced

Applesauce

Many recipes call for butter or other fat sources to add moisture to baked goods. Applesauce is an excellent alternative to add moisture and hold your ingredients together without adding extra fat. Apples are also high in fiber and pectin, two ingredients that help you feel full and satisfied between meals, making them an excellent snack.

1. Heat a medium nonstick pan over medium heat for 5 minutes.

2. Combine all ingredients except oil and apple in a blender, blending until mixed well.

3. Lightly oil the pan, coating all surfaces.

4. Slowly pour ¼ of batter into the pan.

5. When mixture starts to bubble, top with ¼ of apples and flip.

6. Cook 1 more minute, then serve immediately.

Per Serving (1 pancake) | Calories: 386 | Fat: 8 g | Protein: 27 g | Sodium: 646 mg | Fiber: 8 g | Carbohydrates: 55 g | Sugar: 20 g

Chocolate Protein French Toast

French toast is traditionally loaded with calories. This version provides the protein, carbs, and fats you need for a balanced meal.

INGREDIENTS | SERVES 1

Cooking spray
3 large egg whites
½ scoop chocolate protein powder
2 slices whole-grain bread
1 packet stevia
1 teaspoon cinnamon
½ cup sugar-free maple syrup

The Best Bread?

When choosing a bread, look for a whole-grain, multigrain, or sprouted bread. The calories will be similar to white bread, but you'll be getting more fiber and other beneficial nutrients. The high fiber content can also help with feelings of fullness and satiety between meals.

1. Heat a medium skillet over medium-high heat and coat lightly with cooking spray.

2. Whisk together egg whites and protein in a large bowl.

3. Dip bread into egg and protein mixture, coating both sides.

4. Add slices to skillet, cooking 2–3 minutes per side or until golden brown.

5. Remove from skillet; top with stevia, cinnamon, and syrup. Serve immediately.

Per Serving | Calories: 295 | Fat: 2 g | Protein: 29 g | Sodium: 689 mg | Fiber: 3 g | Carbohydrates: 46 g | Sugar: 7 g

Whipped Protein Bowl

When life gets busy, sometimes you don't have time to be cooking fancy breakfasts. This recipe can be assembled in under two minutes for a fast, nutritious meal on the go.

INGREDIENTS | SERVES 1

½ cup fat-free Greek yogurt
1 scoop vanilla whey protein
¼ cup water
1 cup frozen mixed berries
½ cup fat-free whipped cream

1. Combine yogurt, protein, and water in a small bowl, whisking until blended.

2. Let bowl sit in freezer 5 minutes to thicken.

3. Remove from freezer, top with berries and whipped cream, and serve.

Per Serving | Calories: 333 | Fat: 8 g | Protein: 38 g | Sodium: 86 mg | Fiber: 3.5 g | Carbohydrates: 30 g | Sugar: 22 g

Greek Spinach Wrap

This is not only a delicious and easy breakfast; it's also loaded with lean protein and powerful antioxidants to start your day.

INGREDIENTS | SERVES 1

Cooking spray

3 large egg whites

1 cup chopped baby spinach

¼ cup feta cheese

2 tablespoons sun-dried tomatoes, chopped

1 medium whole-wheat tortilla

1. Heat a medium skillet over medium heat and coat lightly with cooking spray.

2. Scramble egg whites and spinach until fully cooked.

3. Add feta cheese and mix well.

4. Spread tomatoes in tortilla, add egg mixture, roll, and serve.

Per Serving | Calories: 175 | Fat: 8.5 g | Protein: 18 g | Sodium: 549 mg | Fiber: 1.5 g | Carbohydrates: 7 g | Sugar: 5 g

The Power of Spinach

Spinach is one of the most nutritious greens you can eat, and it's very mild in flavor. You can add spinach to nearly anything for an added nutrient boost without negatively affecting the taste. It's best to buy spinach fresh whenever possible, as frozen spinach can add significant moisture to a meal as it thaws, throwing off your recipe and food texture.

Island Breakfast Bowl

This is a refreshing and delicious fruit bowl, perfect for a light, energizing start to your day.

INGREDIENTS | SERVES 1

1½ cups frozen pineapple chunks
1 medium banana, sliced
1 cup coconut milk
½ scoop vanilla whey protein
¼ cup coconut flakes

Nuts for Coconuts

In addition to being one of the most delicious fruits on the planet, coconuts provide a good source of healthy fats. The whole fruit is great, but you can also use coconut oil as a healthy fat source. It's perfect for adding flavor, greasing a pan or grill, or adding to smoothies and yogurt for a healthy fat booster. Many stores also sell coconut oil in spray cans, if you want to use it for your baking and cooking.

1. Set aside ¼ cup pineapple and ¼ of sliced banana.

2. Combine all other ingredients in a blender and blend until smooth.

3. Pour in a medium bowl and top with remaining pineapple and banana before serving.

Per Serving | Calories: 819 | Fat: 58 g | Protein: 21 g | Sodium: 58 mg | Fiber: 9 g | Carbohydrates: 70 g | Sugar: 40 g

Southern Baked Avocado and Egg

This dish gives you a nice hit of healthy fats for a hunger-fighting source of sustained energy. It's perfect for low-carb dieting days.

INGREDIENTS | SERVES 4

2 whole medium avocados, cut in half lengthwise and pitted

4 large eggs

1 teaspoon sea salt

1 teaspoon freshly ground black pepper

2 slices bacon, cooked and crumbled

2 tablespoons hot sauce

Start with Fat

Fat is a slow-digesting source of energy and is great for feeling full and avoiding energy crashes. Many people report improved mental functioning when they consume high-fat breakfasts in the morning, so try this kind of breakfast when working on big projects for a boost of brain power. Depending on your goals, you can adjust egg recipes to have more or less fat. Use whole eggs and full-fat cheese if you want more fat or all egg whites and low-fat cheese if you want a meal with less fat.

1. Preheat oven to 350°F.

2. Place avocado halves on a baking sheet and crack 1 egg into each half, using the holes left by the pits. Add yolk first and then as much egg white as you can fit without it spilling over.

3. Season with salt and pepper and bake 20 minutes or until egg whites are solid.

4. Sprinkle bacon on baked avocados, garnish with hot sauce, and serve.

Per Serving | Calories: 251 | Fat: 21 g | Protein: 10 g | Sodium: 937 mg | Fiber: 5 g | Carbohydrates: 7 g | Sugar: 1 g

Low-Carb Southwestern Egg Wrap

By skipping the tortilla, you can use eggs to add healthy fats and proteins to your meal while lowering your carb intake.

INGREDIENTS | SERVES 1

½ tablespoon butter

2 large eggs

1 tablespoon skim milk

2 slices bacon, cooked and crumbled

½ medium avocado, sliced

¼ cup shredded Mexican cheese

½ teaspoon salt

½ teaspoon freshly ground black pepper

½ cup fresh salsa

Make Your Own Salsa

Salsa is an incredibly versatile and low-calorie snack that goes well with anything. You can top meat, eggs, or any Mexican dish with salsa, or enjoy it plain. Store-bought salsas are fine, but it's very easy to make at home, and there are countless recipes. The easiest base recipe is to chop 2 tomatoes, half an onion, 2 tablespoons cilantro, and 1 tablespoon minced garlic. From there, add any flavor enhancers or extra ingredients that you enjoy.

1. Heat a medium skillet over medium-high heat and coat lightly with butter.

2. Mix eggs and milk in a small bowl with a fork and pour into heated pan.

3. Cook 1–2 minutes per side, flipping when edges start to peel off the pan.

4. Plate eggs, and add bacon, avocado, and cheese before rolling into a burrito shape.

5. Season with salt and pepper, top with salsa, and serve.

Per Serving | Calories: 731 | Fat: 60 g | Protein: 32 g | Sodium: 2,916 mg | Fiber: 8 g | Carbohydrates: 19 g | Sugar: 8 g

Cauliflower Toast

If you're following a low-carb plan, cauliflower toast is a great way to replace any bread you may have been eating. It's easy to make, and you can save the leftovers in the refrigerator for several days.

INGREDIENTS | MAKES 6 SLICES

1 medium cauliflower head, chopped or grated
1 large egg
½ cup shredded Cheddar cheese
1 teaspoon garlic salt
1 teaspoon freshly ground black pepper

1. Preheat oven to 425°F. Microwave cauliflower in a large bowl 8–10 minutes.

2. Rinse and drain cauliflower and add egg, cheese, garlic salt, and pepper, mixing well.

3. On a baking sheet lined with parchment paper, divide cauliflower mix into 6 portions and form into your desired shape, spreading the mixture until it is about the size of a small piece of bread, roughly ½" thick.

4. Bake 15–20 minutes until golden brown.

5. Remove from baking sheet and serve with whatever toppings you enjoy.

Per Serving (1 slice) | Calories: 82 | Fat: 5 g | Protein: 6 g | Sodium: 500 mg | Fiber: 2 g | Carbohydrates: 5 g | Sugar: 2 g

Avocado Toast

This combo is perfect for meeting your daily carb quota, and the fat content will help slow down digestion so you don't experience an energy spike and abrupt crash from the toast. For an extra protein boost, you can top this recipe with fried or scrambled eggs.

INGREDIENTS | SERVES 1

1 medium avocado, mashed

1 teaspoon garlic salt

1 teaspoon freshly ground black pepper

2 slices whole-grain bread

1. In a medium bowl, combine avocado, garlic salt, and pepper.

2. Toast bread to desired doneness and spread avocado mixture on each slice before serving.

Per Serving | Calories: 398 | Fat: 24 g | Protein: 8 g | Sodium: 2,621 mg | Fiber: 12 g | Carbohydrates: 43 g | Sugar: 4 g

Superfood Breakfast Bowl

This high-carb recipe is loaded with micronutrients. This is the perfect fuel-up meal for high-activity days, as the carbohydrates and fiber will keep you full while providing electrolytes to keep you hydrated and energized during physical activity.

INGREDIENTS | SERVES 2

½ cup unsweetened plain almond milk

½ teaspoon cinnamon

½ teaspoon vanilla extract

¼ cup uncooked quinoa

1 medium banana, sliced

6 strawberries, sliced

½ cup blueberries

2 teaspoons hemp seeds

1. In a small saucepan, bring almond milk, cinnamon, and vanilla to a boil.

2. Stir in quinoa, reduce to a simmer, and cook 20 minutes or until desired consistency is reached.

3. Top with banana, berries, and hemp seeds. Enjoy warm.

Per Serving | Calories: 200 | Fat: 4 g | Protein: 6 g | Sodium: 43 mg | Fiber: 6 g | Carbohydrates: 38 g | Sugar: 14 g

Breakfast Bake

This recipe is packed with proteins, healthy fats, and flavorful micronutrients from the variety of vegetables it contains.

INGREDIENTS | SERVES 8

1 tablespoon olive oil
2 cups low-fat shredded mozzarella
1 medium red bell pepper, seeded and chopped
2 cups chopped broccoli
4 slices turkey bacon, cooked and crumbled
8 large eggs
4 large egg whites
¼ cup skim milk
2 tablespoons grated Parmesan cheese
½ teaspoon salt
¼ teaspoon freshly ground black pepper

Breakfast for the Week

Making a breakfast bake on Sunday is a great way to prepare for a busy week. This large recipe can be refrigerated and reheated when ready to eat, so you'll have healthy breakfasts ready to go all week long. Try mixing up the vegetables you add to the bake to get a good variety of nutrients week after week.

1. Preheat oven to 375°F.

2. Lightly oil a 9" × 13" glass baking dish and sprinkle half the mozzarella in the bottom.

3. In a medium nonstick pan over medium heat, sauté bell pepper and broccoli 3–4 minutes.

4. Combine vegetables with turkey bacon in a medium bowl and spread mixture over cheese in the dish.

5. In a separate medium bowl combine eggs, egg whites, milk, Parmesan, salt, and black pepper and whisk well.

6. Carefully and evenly pour egg mixture over vegetables and cheese and then top with remaining mozzarella.

7. Bake 30–35 minutes, until a knife inserted into the dish comes out clean. Let stand 5 minutes before serving.

Per Serving | Calories: 223 | Fat: 15 g | Protein: 17 g | Sodium: 562 mg | Fiber: 1 g | Carbohydrates: 4 g | Sugar: 2 g

Maple Pecan Banana Muffins

These low-fat, high-carb muffins are perfect for exercise fuel or recovery. Whether you want an energizing breakfast or a quick pre-workout meal, having these muffins on hand is an easy way to have carbs on the go.

INGREDIENTS | MAKES 12 MUFFINS

1¼ cups whole-wheat flour

¾ teaspoon baking soda

½ teaspoon salt

2 tablespoons unsalted butter, softened

¼ cup brown sugar (or stevia alternative)

2 large egg whites

3 ripe medium bananas

¼ cup pure maple syrup

2 tablespoons unsweetened applesauce

½ teaspoon vanilla extract

⅓ cup crushed pecans

1. Preheat oven to 325°F.

2. Line a 12-cup muffin tin with baking liners.

3. Combine flour, baking soda, and salt in a large bowl and mix well.

4. In a separate large bowl, mix butter and brown sugar until smooth.

5. Add egg whites, bananas, maple syrup, applesauce, and vanilla and mix by hand or with an electric mixer until well blended.

6. Gently stir in flour mixture until combined and then evenly divide into lined muffin cups.

7. Sprinkle muffin tops with pecans and bake 30–35 minutes, until a toothpick inserted into the center comes out clean.

Per Serving (1 muffin) | Calories: 143 | Fat: 5 g | Protein: 3 g | Sodium: 191 mg | Fiber: 2.5 g | Carbohydrates: 25 g | Sugar: 7 g

Asparagus and Swiss Cheese Frittata

This frittata is a quick and good-for-you breakfast that will start your day strong with healthy fats, protein, and green vegetables.

INGREDIENTS | SERVES 4

2 teaspoons butter

½ cup chopped shallots

½ pound asparagus, cooked and chopped

3 large eggs

5 large egg whites

2 tablespoons grated Romano cheese

¼ cup low-fat shredded Swiss cheese

1 tablespoon skim milk

1 teaspoon salt

1 teaspoon freshly ground black pepper

1. Preheat oven to 350°F.

2. Heat butter in a 10-inch cast-iron skillet over medium-low heat. Sauté shallots 5 minutes and then add asparagus.

3. In a separate bowl, combine eggs, egg whites, Romano cheese, Swiss cheese, milk, salt, and pepper.

4. Pour egg mixture over shallots and asparagus in the skillet and continue to cook about 5 minutes.

5. Transfer skillet to oven and cook 16–18 minutes or until frittata is completely cooked though.

Per Serving | Calories: 159 | Fat: 9 g | Protein: 14 g | Sodium: 782 mg | Fiber: 2 g | Carbohydrates: 7 g | Sugar: 3 g

Egg and Cheese Muffins

These portable muffins are easy to eat hot or cold and can be made in large batches and frozen until ready to serve. They are a virtually zero-carb snack with protein and fiber to keep you feeling full all day. If you want to lower the fat, replace the whole eggs with more whites.

INGREDIENTS | MAKES 8 MUFFINS

1 teaspoon olive oil
4 cups chopped broccoli, cooked
4 large eggs
1 cup liquid egg whites
¼ teaspoon salt
¼ teaspoon freshly ground black pepper
¼ cup low-fat shredded Cheddar cheese

Fear Not the Egg

Whole eggs get a bad reputation. Because the yolks are high in cholesterol, many believe that consuming eggs increases bad cholesterol. This is simply not true. Egg yolks contain cholesterol, but some cholesterol is necessary for proper hormonal functioning. The egg yolks are also the most nutritious part of the egg, containing many other beneficial nutrients your body will use.

1. Preheat oven to 350°F.

2. Lightly oil a muffin tin, and divide the broccoli between 8 muffin cups.

3. In a medium bowl, combine eggs, egg whites, salt, and pepper.

4. Pour egg mix into the muffin cups, covering broccoli but leaving about ¼ of each cup empty to allow for rising.

5. Top with Cheddar cheese and bake 15–20 minutes or until fully cooked.

Per Serving (1 muffin) | Calories: 101 | Fat: 5 g | Protein: 9 g | Sodium: 144 mg | Fiber: 3 g | Carbohydrates: 6 g | Sugar: 1 g

Low-Fat Red Velvet Pancakes

This recipe removes most of the fat from traditional pancakes and uses lower-calorie substitutes wherever possible. The pancakes can be served with sugar-free maple syrup and whipped cream or a low-fat cream cheese frosting.

INGREDIENTS | MAKES 10 PANCAKES

1 cup whole-wheat flour

2¼ teaspoons baking powder

½ tablespoon unsweetened cocoa powder

¼ cup stevia

¼ teaspoon salt

1 cup skim milk

1 large egg

1 teaspoon vanilla extract

½ teaspoon red food coloring (optional)

Olive oil to coat the skillet

1. Heat a medium nonstick skillet over medium heat for 5 minutes.

2. Combine flour, baking powder, cocoa powder, stevia, and salt in a large bowl, mixing well.

3. Add milk, egg, vanilla, and red food coloring (if using), and combine until mixed well.

4. Lightly oil the skillet, coating all surfaces.

5. Pour ¼ cup batter into the skillet. Flip after 2–3 minutes or when pancake starts to bubble, and cook for another minute on the second side.

Per Serving (1 pancake) | Calories: 61 | Fat: 1 g | Protein: 3 g | Sodium: 186 mg | Fiber: 1 g | Carbohydrates: 15 g | Sugar: 1 g

Banana Pancakes

This recipe uses a banana to add moisture and nutrition. In addition to being a great source of natural sugars and healthy carbohydrates, bananas are loaded with potassium, an important electrolyte to keep you hydrated while you exercise.

INGREDIENTS | MAKES 12 PANCAKES

1 cup whole-wheat flour
2 teaspoons baking powder
¼ teaspoon salt
¼ teaspoon cinnamon
1 cup skim milk
3 large egg whites
2 teaspoons olive oil
1 teaspoon vanilla extract
1 large ripe banana, mashed
Olive oil to coat the skillet

1. Heat a medium nonstick skillet over medium heat for 5 minutes.

2. Mix flour, baking powder, salt, and cinnamon in a large bowl.

3. In a separate large bowl, add milk, egg whites, oil, vanilla, and banana and mix until smooth, then combine with the dry ingredients.

4. Lightly oil the skillet, coating all surfaces.

5. Pour ¼ cup batter into the skillet, flipping after 2–3 minutes or when pancake starts to bubble, and cook the second side for an additional minute.

Per Serving (1 pancake) | Calories: 65 | Fat: 1 g | Protein: 3 g | Sodium: 153 mg | Fiber: 1 g | Carbohydrates: 11 g | Sugar: 3 g

Peanut Butter and Jelly Yogurt Bowl

This fast and easy breakfast combines all the flavors of your favorite childhood lunch, giving you a healthy dose of protein, fats, and carbs. It can be assembled in minutes and is perfect for busy mornings when you don't have time to make a hot meal.

INGREDIENTS | SERVES 1

6 ounces fat-free, plain Greek yogurt
4 teaspoons reduced-sugar grape jelly
1 tablespoon natural peanut butter
1 teaspoon unsalted peanuts
½ cup grapes, washed and cut in half

1. Combine yogurt, jelly, and peanut butter in a small bowl and mix.

2. Top with peanuts and grapes and serve immediately.

Per Serving | Calories: 308 | Fat: 10.5 g | Protein: 22 g | Sodium: 131 mg | Fiber: 2 g | Carbohydrates: 35 g | Sugar: 30 g

CHAPTER 7

Lunch

Cilantro Chicken and Avocado Burritos

If you have precooked chicken available, this recipe can be assembled in minutes. Use grilled or roasted chicken strips from the store or make your own using your favorite chicken recipe.

INGREDIENTS | SERVES 4

1 pound chicken, cooked and shredded

1 medium avocado, diced

1 cup shredded Mexican cheese

1 cup salsa verde

½ cup sour cream

4 tablespoons chopped cilantro

4 large tortillas

1. Equally distribute all ingredients between tortillas.

2. Roll up tortillas to form burritos and serve.

Per Serving | Calories: 497 | Fat: 26 g | Protein: 35 g | Sodium: 632 mg | Fiber: 4 g | Carbohydrates: 31 g | Sugar: 4 g

Rotate Your Chicken

These burritos can be assembled with any sort of precooked chicken (served warm or cold). Many grocery stores sell precooked chicken, either whole or already sliced. If you're running short on time, this is an excellent shortcut. You can use it plain or add any seasoning or sauce you want to keep the flavor interesting.

Protein Pizza "Muffins"

These are easy to make in large batches and are ready to grab and go whenever you want pizza flavor without the pizza calories.

INGREDIENTS | MAKES 12 MUFFINS

18 slices turkey pepperoni, chopped
9 large eggs
2 cloves garlic, minced
1 cup chopped sun-dried tomatoes
3 teaspoons Italian seasoning
1 teaspoon onion powder
½ teaspoon salt

1. Preheat oven to 400°F.

2. Lightly grease a 12-cup muffin tin.

3. In a large bowl, whisk together all ingredients.

4. Pour mixture into the muffin tin, filling each cup ¾ full.

5. Bake 15 minutes or until muffins have set and begun to brown.

6. Remove, allow to cool 5 minutes, and serve.

Per Serving (1 muffin) | Calories: 74 | Fat: 4 g | Protein: 6 g | Sodium: 216 mg | Fiber: 1 g | Carbohydrates: 3 g | Sugar: 2 g

California Roll in a Bowl

The California roll may be the most popular sushi roll in America, and the ingredients are quite simple. If you want a sushi fix but don't want to learn how to roll it yourself, this bowl is a quick and easy way to enjoy some fresh California roll.

INGREDIENTS | SERVES 2

2 cups cooked white rice

½ cup chopped imitation crab

½ medium cucumber, peeled and chopped

½ medium avocado, sliced

1 sheet dried seaweed, crumbled

1 tablespoon toasted sesame seeds

¼ cup soy sauce

¼ cup rice vinegar

¼ cup pickled sushi ginger (optional)

1. Combine all ingredients except soy sauce, vinegar, and ginger in a large bowl and mix well.

2. Evenly divide mixture into 2 serving bowls.

3. In a separate container, mix soy sauce and vinegar.

4. Drizzle sauce over rice mixture, top with ginger if desired, and serve.

Per Serving | Calories: 437 | Fat: 8 g | Protein: 13 g | Sodium: 2,450 mg | Fiber: 4 g | Carbohydrates: 78 g | Sugar: 14 g

Shrimp Ceviche Salad

This is a quick and easy dish that packs lean protein and healthy fats. You can enjoy this salad as is or, if you want some extra carbs, try serving it with tortilla chips for dipping.

INGREDIENTS | SERVES 2

1 large avocado, diced

2 green onion stalks, chopped

1 (4-ounce) can salad shrimp

1 medium tomato, diced

3 tablespoons chopped cilantro

1 teaspoon salt

1 teaspoon freshly ground black pepper

½ medium lime

1. Add all ingredients, except lime, to a large bowl. Gently toss until mixed well, being careful not to smash the avocado chunks too much.

2. Divide into 2 medium bowls, top each with a squeeze of lime juice, and serve.

Per Serving | Calories: 223 | Fat: 14 g | Protein: 14 g | Sodium: 1,663 mg | Fiber: 8 g | Carbohydrates: 16 g | Sugar: 3 g

Canned Seafood

While canned seafoods like tuna, crab, or shrimp may not be quite as tasty and nutritious as their fresh alternatives, they are a quick and easy source of ready-to-go protein. Try not to get all of your seafood from a can, but when you want something convenient and quick, like in this recipe, canned seafood is an excellent option to have around.

Burrito Bowl with Spicy Protein Sauce

This is a low-calorie, protein-packed alternative to a popular Mexican lunch.
You can substitute ground beef instead of ground turkey for some extra fats.

INGREDIENTS | SERVES 4

1 cup uncooked jasmine rice

1½ cups water

1½ teaspoons salt, divided

1 pound lean ground turkey

1 tablespoon taco seasoning

2 tablespoons hot sauce

¼ cup plain Greek yogurt

1 (15-ounce) can black beans, drained and rinsed

2 medium avocados, diced

Why Avocado?

Avocados are a very good source of potassium and monounsaturated fat (the good kind of fat). They can be used for much more than guacamole, as this recipe shows. If you want less fat, you can always leave out the avocado.

1. In a medium saucepan, combine rice, water, and ½ teaspoon salt. Bing to a boil. Stir once, cover, and reduce heat to low. Simmer 18–20 minutes. Remove from heat and fluff with fork. Set aside.

2. Brown turkey in a medium skillet over medium heat until no longer pink. Strain excess fat and season turkey with taco seasoning and remaining salt.

3. In a small bowl, combine hot sauce and yogurt, mixing well.

4. Scoop rice into 4 serving bowls, and top with turkey, beans, and avocado. Drizzle with spicy yogurt sauce and serve.

Per Serving | Calories: 564 | Fat: 21 g | Protein: 34 g | Sodium: 1,607 mg | Fiber: 10 g | Carbohydrates: 61 g | Sugar: 4 g

Chicken and Kale Caesar Salad

This spin on a common salad increases the nutrition with the inclusion of kale,
one of the most nutritious greens available.

INGREDIENTS | SERVES 4

¼ cup freshly grated Parmesan, plus more for serving

¼ cup plain Greek yogurt

¼ cup lemon juice

½ teaspoon Worcestershire sauce

3 tablespoons olive oil, divided

1 clove garlic, minced

1 pound boneless, skinless chicken breast

½ teaspoon salt

½ teaspoon freshly ground black pepper

4 cups kale

The Power of Kale

Kale is a superfood, and considered one of the most nutrient-dense foods on earth. It's an excellent source of vitamin K, vitamin C, vitamin A, and many other vitamins and minerals. Any time you're eating greens, adding kale to the mix is a great way to increase the nutritional value of your meal.

1. Dressing: combine Parmesan, yogurt, lemon juice, Worcestershire sauce, 2 tablespoons olive oil, and garlic in a food processor and mix well.

2. Heat a medium skillet over medium heat 5 minutes.

3. Season chicken with salt and pepper.

4. Lightly oil the pan with remaining olive oil, coating all surfaces.

5. Place chicken in skillet and cook 6–8 minutes per side or until fully cooked through, then shred once fully cooked.

6. Gather 4 separate serving bowls, placing 1 cup kale in each. Divide chicken between bowls, top with dressing, and serve.

Per Serving | Calories: 280 | Fat: 16 g | Protein: 30 g | Sodium: 460 mg | Fiber: 1 g | Carbohydrates: 4 g | Sugar: 1 g

Asian Salmon Salad

This sesame-ginger infused, Asian-inspired salad is an excellent source of healthy fats to supercharge your day. It works best with salmon, but any fish can be used.

INGREDIENTS | SERVES 4

2 tablespoons soy sauce

1" piece ginger, chopped

1 clove garlic, minced

2 tablespoons chopped green onions

¼ cup vegetable oil

3 tablespoons white vinegar

1 tablespoon sesame oil

1 tablespoon olive oil

4 salmon fillets (about 2 pounds total)

2 teaspoons salt

2 teaspoons freshly ground black pepper

4 cups mixed greens

1. Dressing: combine soy sauce, ginger, garlic, onions, vegetable oil, vinegar, and sesame oil in a food processor, blending until smooth.

2. Add olive oil to a cast-iron skillet or nonstick pan and heat over medium heat. Season salmon with salt and pepper and cook 4–5 minutes per side, then flake into pieces.

3. Gather 4 separate serving bowls, 1 cup greens in each. Top with salmon and drizzle with dressing before serving.

Per Serving | Calories: 524 | Fat: 35 g | Protein: 46 g | Sodium: 1,726 mg | Fiber: 1 g | Carbohydrates: 4 g | Sugar: 0 g

Buffalo Chicken Mini Wraps

These bite-sized wraps are the perfect lunch. Once prepared, you can grab one anytime you need it, and you can wrap the mix in lettuce leaves instead of tortillas if you don't want the carbs.

INGREDIENTS | MAKES 15 WRAPS

3 large boneless, skinless chicken breasts, cut into ½" cubes

¾ cup Frank's RedHot Original Cayenne Pepper Sauce, divided

Nonstick cooking spray

1 medium avocado, diced

15 mini tortillas

½ cup low-fat ranch dressing

1. Place the chicken in a large bowl or resealable bag. Pour ½ cup hot sauce over chicken and marinate 1–2 hours in the refrigerator.

2. When ready to cook, heat a large skillet over medium heat, lightly coat with cooking spray, and cook chicken 10–12 minutes or until fully cooked through.

3. Add remaining hot sauce to cooked chicken, toss, and let cool 5 minutes.

4. Equally divide chicken and avocado between tortillas, drizzle with dressing, and serve.

Per Serving (1 wrap) | Calories: 170 | Fat: 5 g | Protein: 14 g | Sodium: 728 mg | Fiber: 1 g | Carbohydrates: 16 g | Sugar: 2 g

Lemon-Parsley Bean Salad

This meat-free dish provides protein and fiber from the beans, with a refreshing, Lebanese-inspired flavor.

INGREDIENTS | SERVES 6

¼ cup olive oil

¼ cup lemon juice

3 cloves garlic, minced

¾ teaspoon salt

2 (14-ounce) cans red kidney beans, drained and rinsed

1 (14-ounce) can chickpeas, drained and rinsed

1 small red onion, peeled and diced

2 stalks celery, chopped

1 medium cucumber, peeled and diced

¾ cup chopped fresh parsley

2 tablespoons chopped dill

1. Dressing: whisk together oil, lemon juice, garlic, and salt until emulsified.

2. Combine kidney beans, chickpeas, onion, celery, cucumber, parsley, and dill in a medium bowl, mixing well.

3. Mix the bean mixture and dressing together, tossing to combine. Divide into 6 servings.

Per Serving | Calories: 785 | Fat: 14 g | Protein: 45 g | Sodium: 363 mg | Fiber: 42 g | Carbohydrates: 125 g | Sugar: 12 g

Tuna Salad

This protein-packed recipe is perfect for when you need a quick meal. You can enjoy it as a traditional sandwich, a tortilla wrap, or plain if you're watching your carbs.

INGREDIENTS | SERVES 4

2 (6-ounce) cans tuna packed in water
¼ teaspoon freshly ground black pepper
1 tablespoon olive oil
½ small red onion, peeled and thinly sliced
¼ cup roughly chopped kalamata olives

1. Drain and rinse tuna, removing any excess water and fat.

2. In a medium bowl, combine tuna, pepper, oil, onion, and olives. Mix well and enjoy.

Per Serving | Calories: 208 | Fat: 10 g | Protein: 25 g | Sodium: 351 mg | Fiber: 0 g | Carbohydrates: 3 g | Sugar: 0 g

Does Canned Tuna Have Healthy Fats?

You may see advertising on tuna cans that it is high in omega-3, a good fat. While this is true of whole tuna, it is not always true with canned tuna. Look at the nutrition label and get tuna with higher fat if you want the omega-3 fatty acids. If they advertise high omega-3, but a serving only has .5 grams of fat, you aren't really getting many good fats.

Turkey Reuben Sandwiches

A Reuben is traditionally a high-calorie meal, but this version drastically lowers the high fat content typically found in Reubens.

INGREDIENTS | SERVES 2

1 tablespoon olive oil
4 ounces sliced turkey
2 slices reduced-fat Swiss cheese
½ cup sauerkraut, drained
¼ cup fat-free Thousand Island dressing
4 slices rye bread

Sauerkraut and Your Gut

Fermented foods like sauerkraut provide an excellent source of live probiotics, which are essential for a healthy gut. Having the proper balance of good bacteria, which are found in fermented foods like sauerkraut, kimchi, and certain kinds of yogurt, will help maintain a healthy gut environment. A healthy gut strengthens your immune system and keeps your digestive system functioning.

1. Heat oil in a nonstick skillet over medium heat.

2. While pan heats, evenly divide turkey, cheese, sauerkraut, and dressing between the slices of rye bread, stacking two with toppings, then topping with the remaining two slices.

3. Cook sandwich in skillet 3–4 minutes per side, until bread is toasted and warm, then serve.

Per Serving | Calories: 403 | Fat: 15 g | Protein: 23 g | Sodium: 1,502 mg | Fiber: 6 g | Carbohydrates: 43 g | Sugar: 9 g

Turkey and Spinach Focaccia Sandwich

This sandwich provides lean protein from the turkey, as well as micronutrients from the spinach and tomatoes. For added flavor and texture, lightly toast the focaccia bread slices before preparing.

INGREDIENTS | SERVES 2

2 tablespoons low-fat mayonnaise

2 tablespoons chopped fresh basil

2 tablespoons sun-dried tomatoes

¼ teaspoon crushed red pepper

4 slices focaccia bread

8 ounces sliced turkey

1 cup spinach leaves

1. In a small bowl, mix mayonnaise, basil, tomatoes, and crushed red pepper. Divide the mixture in half.

2. Build sandwiches by layering the spread, turkey, and spinach leaves.

Per Serving | Calories: 421 | Fat: 13 g | Protein: 25 g | Sodium: 1,679 mg | Fiber: 1 g | Carbohydrates: 52 g | Sugar: 3 g

Which Bread Should You Choose?

In terms of pure calories, there isn't a huge variety among bread manufacturers. You'll likely find most slices range from 80–140 calories. For maximum health, however, a sprouted whole-grain bread will be full of fiber and beneficial nutrients.

Chipotle Lime Cod Fillets

This recipe takes a bit longer to prepare, but it can be made in bulk and reheated in minutes. When topped with the creamy avocado sauce, this is a delicious meal full of healthy fats.

INGREDIENTS | SERVES 4

Fish

1 canned chipotle pepper

2 tablespoons adobo sauce

¼ cup salsa

1 tablespoon lime juice

4 (6-ounce) cod fillets

Sauce

1 small avocado, diced

¼ cup low-fat sour cream

1 tablespoon lime juice

1 teaspoon salt

1 teaspoon freshly ground black pepper

3 tablespoons skim milk

1. Preheat oven to 375°F.

2. In a blender, combine chipotle pepper, adobo sauce, salsa, and lime.

3. Brush both sides of fillets with chipotle mix and place in a lightly oiled 9" × 9" glass baking dish.

4. Bake fillets 20–25 minutes, turning once halfway through. Fish is done when it flakes easily with a fork.

5. While fish bakes, place avocado, sour cream, lime juice, salt, and pepper in a blender and blend until smooth.

6. Transfer to a small bowl, stir in skim milk, and set aside.

7. When fish is cooked, top with avocado sauce and serve.

Per Serving | Calories: 293 | Fat: 9 g | Protein: 44 g | Sodium: 1,684 mg | Fiber: 5 g | Carbohydrates: 9 g | Sugar: 4 g

Egg Salad

*Egg salad is a very versatile dish that can be served on a sandwich, added to a salad,
or enjoyed as a side dish that's loaded with fat and protein.*

INGREDIENTS | SERVES 4

8 large eggs

½ cup low-fat mayonnaise

1 teaspoon mustard

¼ cup chopped green onion

¼ teaspoon salt

¼ teaspoon freshly ground black pepper

¼ teaspoon paprika

1. Place eggs in a medium saucepan and add cold water until eggs are covered by 1 inch of water.

2. Bring water to a boil, then immediately remove pan from heat. Cover and let eggs cook 10–12 minutes, then immediately drain and cool under running cold water.

3. Peel eggs, chop, and mix with mayonnaise, mustard, onion, and seasonings.

Per Serving | Calories: 176 | Fat: 12 g | Protein: 13 g | Sodium: 559 mg | Fiber: 0 g | Carbohydrates: 5 g | Sugar: 3 g

Avocado, Chickpea, and Quinoa Salad

*Avocado and chickpea are two excellent sources of healthy fats,
and quinoa is one of the healthiest grains available.*

INGREDIENTS | SERVES 4

1 cup cooked quinoa

1 (15-ounce) can chickpeas

2 tablespoons minced red onion

2 tablespoons minced cilantro

4 tablespoons lime juice

¼ teaspoon salt

¼ teaspoon freshly ground black pepper

1 cup diced cucumber

1 medium avocado, diced

1. Combine all ingredients except cucumber and avocado in a large bowl.

2. When ready to eat, mix in cucumber and avocado and serve immediately.

Per Serving | Calories: 215 | Fat: 8 g | Protein: 8 g | Sodium: 163 mg | Fiber: 7 g | Carbohydrates: 30 g | Sugar: 4 g

Potato Soup

*This hearty meal combines all the flavors of a traditional baked potato.
It is perfect for a warm and filling lunch and is great on a cold or rainy day.*

INGREDIENTS | MAKES 5 CUPS

2 medium russet potatoes
1 small head cauliflower, chopped
1½ cups fat-free chicken broth
1½ cups skim milk
½ cup light sour cream
½ cup low-fat shredded Cheddar cheese
6 tablespoons chopped chives
1 teaspoon salt
1 teaspoon freshly ground black pepper
3 slices bacon, cooked and crumbled

1. Preheat oven to 400°F.

2. Bake potatoes 1 hour. Remove and dice.

3. Steam cauliflower over boiling water or in a steamer 5 minutes.

4. Combine potatoes, broth, and milk in a medium saucepan and bring to a boil before adding cauliflower.

5. Lower heat to a simmer, then using a handheld mixer, blend until potatoes are completely softened.

6. Add sour cream, cheese, chives, salt, and pepper and simmer 10 minutes, stirring frequently.

7. Garnish with crumbled bacon before serving.

Per Serving (1 cup) | Calories: 271 | Fat: 13 g | Protein: 13 g | Sodium: 996 mg | Fiber: 4 g | Carbohydrates: 28 g | Sugar: 7 g

Pizza Flatbreads

This is a delicious and fresh French-style flatbread with less fat and more flavor than a traditional pizza.

INGREDIENTS | SERVES 4

1 whole French bread baguette

1 cup low-fat shredded mozzarella cheese

2 medium tomatoes, thinly sliced

1 tablespoon chopped basil

1 tablespoon balsamic glaze

1. Preheat oven to broil.

2. Cut bread in half lengthwise, then cut both halves across, making 4 flatbread portions. Place flatbreads on a baking sheet.

3. Top each piece with ¼ cup cheese and broil until cheese is melted and starts to brown.

4. Remove, top with tomato and basil, drizzle with balsamic glaze, and serve.

Per Serving (1 flatbread) | Calories: 254 | Fat: 6 g | Protein: 15 g | Sodium: 588 mg | Fiber: 2 g | Carbohydrates: 37 g | Sugar: 5 g

Buffalo Chicken Baked Nuggets

This buffalo-wing-flavored meal removes most of the fat from fried buffalo wings, giving you a spicy and delicious lunch. Enjoy them as they are or serve with a side salad. You could also serve them with low-fat ranch or blue cheese if desired.

INGREDIENTS | MAKES 40 NUGGETS

½ teaspoon garlic powder

½ teaspoon paprika

½ teaspoon chili powder

⅛ teaspoon freshly ground black pepper

¼ cup panko bread crumbs

2 tablespoons Frank's RedHot Original Cayenne Pepper Sauce

2 teaspoons olive oil

1 pound boneless, skinless chicken breast, cut into 40 small bite-sized pieces

1. Preheat oven to 425°F.

2. Combine garlic powder, paprika, chili powder, pepper, and bread crumbs in a medium bowl and mix well.

3. In a separate medium bowl, combine hot sauce and oil until well blended.

4. Dip chicken pieces in sauce, roll in crumbs, and place on a lightly oiled baking sheet.

5. Bake 12–15 minutes or until golden brown, removing halfway through to turn over.

Per Serving (10 nuggets) | Calories: 171 | Fat: 5 g | Protein: 26 g | Sodium: 349 mg | Fiber: 0 g | Carbohydrates: 4 g | Sugar: 0 g

CHAPTER 8

Vegetarian and Vegan

Pesto Chili

This recipe contains a variety of beans to help make sure you get as many different essential amino acids and proteins in your diet as possible.

INGREDIENTS | SERVES 4

¼ cup olive oil, divided

2 medium carrots, peeled diced

1 small yellow onion, chopped

1 (15-ounce) can diced tomatoes

1 teaspoon salt

1 teaspoon freshly ground black pepper

2 cups water

1 (15-ounce) can chickpeas, drained and rinsed

1 (15-ounce) can cannellini beans, drained and rinsed

1 (15-ounce) can kidney beans, drained and rinsed

½ cup pesto

1. Add 1 tablespoon oil, carrots, and onion to a large saucepan over high heat and cook 3–5 minutes or until carrots are tender.

2. Stir in tomatoes, salt, pepper, and water and bring to a boil. Add chickpeas and other cans of beans, cooking until heated through (about 3 minutes).

3. Divide into 4 equal portions, top with pesto, and serve.

Per Serving | Calories: 537 | Fat: 39 g | Protein: 11 g | Sodium: 1,209 mg | Fiber: 12 g | Carbohydrates: 37 g | Sugar: 6 g

Mix Your Beans for Proper Protein

One of the biggest challenges with following a vegan or vegetarian diet can be getting adequate protein. Even if your goal isn't to build muscle, you need protein to live and function. While beans contain some protein, they don't necessarily have all the essential amino acids you need to get in your diet. Combining bean sources is a good way to make sure you're getting a variety of amino acids.

Linguine and Caper Sauce

This traditional Mediterranean-style pasta is simple to prepare and can be made in bulk in order to have reheated meals throughout the week.

INGREDIENTS | SERVES 6

1 tablespoon olive oil

2 cloves garlic, minced

¼ teaspoon red pepper flakes

1 (26-ounce) jar marinara sauce

1 (3.5-ounce) jar capers, chopped

½ cup chopped fresh parsley

½ teaspoon lemon zest

1 (16-ounce) package linguine

1. Combine oil, garlic, and red pepper flakes in a large saucepan over medium heat and cook 2 minutes until garlic becomes fragrant.

2. Stir in marinara, capers, parsley, and lemon zest, then reduce heat to low and simmer 15 minutes.

3. While sauce is simmering, prepare linguine according to the package directions.

4. Combine pasta and sauce, tossing until mixed well, and serve.

Per Serving | Calories: 364 | Fat: 5 g | Protein: 12 g | Sodium: 900 mg | Fiber: 5 g | Carbohydrates: 66 g | Sugar: 9 g

Avocado Southwestern Salad

This filling, Southwestern-style salad is packed with healthy fats from the avocado and beans and makes the perfect side dish or stand-alone meal.

INGREDIENTS | SERVES 4

¼ cup olive oil

¼ cup lime juice

½ teaspoon ground cumin

1 teaspoon salt

1 teaspoon freshly ground black pepper

2 bags (about 12 cups) romaine lettuce

2 medium avocados, cubed

1 (15.5-ounce) can pinto beans, drained and rinsed

1 cup cooked corn kernels

½ medium red onion, peeled and diced

½ cup chopped fresh cilantro

1. Dressing: whisk together oil, lime juice, cumin, salt, and pepper until emulsified.

2. Toss lettuce, avocados, beans, corn, onion, and cilantro in a large bowl.

3. Mix dressing with salad and serve.

Per Serving | Calories: 274 | Fat: 15 g | Protein: 8 g | Sodium: 882 mg | Fiber: 9 g | Carbohydrates: 32 g | Sugar: 5 g

Pasta with Pesto and Olive Sauce

This light and healthy dish uses fresh herbs and spices to make a very simple, low-fat recipe. If you want to get your carbs in without feeling weighed down, this is the light meal recipe for you.

INGREDIENTS | SERVES 4

1 (16-ounce) package spaghetti
½ cup reserved pasta water
2 cloves garlic
¼ cup olive oil
¼ cup green olives
¼ cup fresh parsley
¼ cup fresh basil
¼ cup black olives
½ teaspoon salt

1. Cook the spaghetti al dente according to package directions and drain, reserving ½ cup pasta water.

2. To make the pesto, combine garlic, olive oil, green olives, parsley, and basil in a blender and blend thoroughly.

3. Transfer pesto to a large saucepan and heat 2 minutes over medium heat until warm.

4. Add spaghetti, black olives, salt, and reserved water to the saucepan and continue cooking until water is absorbed and spaghetti is heated. Serve immediately.

Per Serving | Calories: 320 | Fat: 17 g | Protein: 7 g | Sodium: 418 mg | Fiber: 3 g | Carbohydrates: 36 g | Sugar: 1 g

Bump Up the Protein with Meat Substitutes

If you're looking to add more protein to meatless dishes, such as this pasta dish, consider adding tofu or tempeh. They are alternatives to protein derived from the soybean, and are an easy way to add some extra protein to your meals, replacing traditional proteins like seafood or meat.

Quinoa and Mushroom Protein Burger

Not only are mushrooms full of important vitamins and minerals, but they also generally have more protein than other vegetables. These delicious burgers are easy to prepare and provide a big hit of protein. Enjoy these burgers as is or serve on a bun with your favorite toppings.

INGREDIENTS | SERVES 4

4 medium portobello mushroom caps, chopped

1 clove garlic, minced

2 tablespoons canola oil, divided

1 teaspoon salt

¼ teaspoon freshly ground black pepper

¼ cup chopped red onion

3 green onions, chopped

2 teaspoons rice wine vinegar

1 cup cooked quinoa

¼ cup cornstarch

Quinoa, the Complete Protein

On a vegetarian diet, it's very important to ensure you are getting complete protein sources that have all the amino acids you need. Quinoa is one of the most complete protein sources in the plant world and should be a staple in your diet.

1. Preheat oven to 375°F.

2. In 9" × 9" glass baking dish, combine mushrooms, garlic, 1 tablespoon oil, salt, and pepper, mixing well.

3. Bake 20 minutes to tenderize mushrooms. Remove from oven and allow to cool. (Dish can be placed in the refrigerator to speed cooling.)

4. Combine mushroom mix, red onion, green onion, and vinegar in a blender, mixing until smooth.

5. Transfer mixture to a large bowl, stirring in quinoa and cornstarch to thicken. Cover and refrigerator at least 2 hours.

6. When ready to eat, form mixture into 4 burger patties and cook in a lightly oiled nonstick skillet over medium heat 5–7 minutes per side.

Per Serving (1 burger) | Calories: 175 | Fat: 8 g | Protein: 4 g | Sodium: 595 mg | Fiber: 3 g | Carbohydrates: 22 g | Sugar: 3 g

Black Bean Soup

This soup requires a slow cooker, but leftovers can be stored in the refrigerator and reheated whenever you need an easy, protein-packed lunch.

INGREDIENTS | SERVES 6

2 tablespoons olive oil

2 medium carrots, chopped and peeled

2 stalks celery, chopped

1 medium onion, peeled and chopped

¼ cup tomato paste

3 cloves garlic, minced

1½ teaspoons ground cumin

3 (15-ounce) cans black beans, drained and rinsed

1 cup frozen or canned corn

3 cups vegetable broth

1. Heat oil in a medium skillet over medium-high heat.

2. Add carrots, celery, and onion to the pan and cook 5 minutes, stirring occasionally.

3. Stir in tomato paste, garlic, and cumin and continue to cook 2 minutes, stirring frequently.

4. In a large slow cooker (at least 4 quarts), combine skillet mixture with beans, corn, and broth. Cook on high 4 hours.

5. Serve warm or allow to cool and refrigerate for later.

Per Serving | Calories: 293 | Fat: 7 g | Protein: 14 g | Sodium: 1,512 mg | Fiber: 12 g | Carbohydrates: 44 g | Sugar: 11 g

Spicy Ranch Chili

This chili has a Southwestern spicy kick, perfect for warming up your cold winter evenings. Like the other chilis and soups in this chapter, this recipe is easy to prepare in bulk and save for later.

INGREDIENTS | SERVES 6

1 (28-ounce) can diced tomatoes, with liquid

1 (15-ounce) can white beans, drained and rinsed

1 (15-ounce) can chili beans, with liquid

1 small onion, peeled and diced

1 (1.25-ounce) package taco seasoning

1 (1-ounce) package ranch dressing mix

¼ cup hot sauce

1 (12-ounce) package vegetarian burger crumbles

1. Combine all ingredients except burger crumbles in a large saucepan and bring to a boil.

2. Reduce to a gentle simmer and stir in burger crumbles.

3. Simmer 10 minutes to heat burger crumbles and serve warm.

Per Serving | Calories: 334 | Fat: 2 g | Protein: 21 g | Sodium: 1,153 mg | Fiber: 17 g | Carbohydrates: 59 g | Sugar: 11 g

Meatless Cheddar Squash Casserole

This casserole provides important nutrients and fiber from the squash, as well as protein from the milk, cheese, and eggs.

INGREDIENTS | SERVES 10

4 cups sliced summer squash
½ cup chopped onion
½ cup water
35 buttery round crackers, crushed
1 cup shredded Cheddar cheese
2 large eggs
¾ cup skim milk
1 teaspoon salt
½ teaspoon freshly ground black pepper
¼ cup unsalted butter, melted

1. Preheat oven to 400°F.

2. Place squash, onion, and water in a large skillet over medium-high heat and cover. Cook 5 minutes or until squash is tender, then drain and set aside.

3. In a medium bowl, combine cracker and cheese until well blended.

4. Stir half the cracker mixture into cooked squash and onions, mixing well.

5. In a separate medium bowl, whisk eggs and milk until well blended. Add to cracker and squash mixture, along with salt, pepper, and melted butter, mixing well.

6. Spread into a greased 9" × 13" glass baking dish, and top with remaining half of cracker and cheese mix.

7. Bake 25 minutes or until lightly browned, then serve.

Per Serving | Calories: 184 | Fat: 13 g | Protein: 7 g | Sodium: 423 mg | Fiber: 1 g | Carbohydrates: 10 g | Sugar: 3 g

Chickpea Salad

This quick and easy chickpea salad can be enjoyed on a sandwich, in a wrap, or on top of a salad.

INGREDIENTS | SERVES 4

1 (19-ounce) can chickpeas, drained and rinsed

1 stalk celery, chopped

½ medium onion, peeled and chopped

1 tablespoon mayonnaise

1 tablespoon lemon juice

1 teaspoon dried dill

1. In a medium bowl mash chickpeas with a fork.

2. Add all other ingredients, mix well, and refrigerate until ready to eat.

Per Serving | Calories: 125 | Fat: 4.2 g | Protein: 5.2 g | Sodium: 33 mg | Fiber: 4.7 g | Carbohydrates: 17.4 g | Sugar: 3.5 g

Zucchini and Potato Bake

Potatoes are full of important nutrients and are a very filling source of carbohydrates. Combined with zucchini, this nutritious and tasty recipe will keep you full for hours.

INGREDIENTS | SERVES 4

2 medium zucchini, sliced

4 medium potatoes, peeled and cut into large chunks

1 medium red bell pepper, seeded and chopped

1 clove garlic, minced

½ cup bread crumbs

¼ cup olive oil

1 teaspoon paprika

1 teaspoon salt

1 teaspoon freshly ground black pepper

1. Preheat oven to 400°F.

2. In a medium baking pan, toss all ingredients together, spreading evenly over the pan.

3. Bake 1 hour or until potatoes are tender, stirring occasionally.

Per Serving | Calories: 349.65 | Fat: 14.9 g | Protein: 7 g | Sodium: 710 mg | Fiber: 7.6 g | Carbohydrates: 48 g | Sugar: 7 g

Vegetable and Tortilla Soup

This soup is brimming with a variety of vegetables that provide many important vitamins and minerals. For an extra kick, serve with your favorite hot sauce.

INGREDIENTS | SERVES 12

2 tablespoons vegetable oil

1 (16-ounce) package frozen stir-fry mix

2 cloves garlic, minced

3 tablespoons ground cumin

1 (28-ounce) can crushed tomatoes

3 (4-ounce) cans chopped green chile peppers, drained

4 (14-ounce) cans vegetable broth

1 (11-ounce) can whole kernel corn

12 ounces whole-grain tortilla chips

1. Heat oil in a large saucepan over medium heat. Add stir-fry, garlic, and cumin and cook 5 minutes, stirring frequently. Add tomatoes, peppers, and broth.

2. Bring soup to a boil, then reduce to a simmer and continue cooking 30 minutes.

3. Mix corn into soup and cook an additional 5 minutes.

4. Fill each bowl halfway with tortilla chips, top with soup, and serve.

Per Serving | Calories: 137 | Fat: 3.87 g | Protein: 3.6 g | Sodium: 499 mg | Fiber: 3.5 g | Carbohydrates: 24.85 g | Sugar: 5 g

Broiled Tomato Sandwich

This quick sandwich combines fresh tomatoes and an herb spread for a delicious, nontraditional, healthy sandwich.

INGREDIENTS | SERVES 2

2 tablespoons olive oil

2 tablespoons balsamic vinegar

1 large tomato, sliced

3 tablespoons reduced-fat mayonnaise

½ teaspoon dried parsley

¼ teaspoon dried oregano

¼ teaspoon freshly ground black pepper

3 tablespoons grated vegetarian Parmesan cheese, divided

4 slices sprouted or whole-grain bread, lightly toasted

Tomatoes for Health

Tomatoes are a very powerful and nutritious food that should be included in your diet on a regular basis. In addition to being loaded with micronutrients, tomatoes can improve your heart health, vision health, and can act as an anticarcinogen, which means they reduce the risk of developing cancer from environmental toxins.

1. Preheat oven to broil.

2. Add olive oil and vinegar to a small bowl and whisk well.

3. Add tomatoes, cover, and marinate 30–60 minutes.

4. In a separate small bowl, mix mayonnaise, parsley, oregano, pepper, and 2 teaspoons Parmesan.

5. Place bread slices on a baking sheet and evenly spread mayonnaise mixture over each slice, topping 2 of the slices with the marinated tomatoes. Place remaining 2 bread slices on top of tomatoes, mayonnaise side down.

6. Broil 5 minutes or until cheese turns golden brown. Serve immediately.

Per Serving | Calories: 339 | Fat: 32 g | Protein: 4.7 g | Sodium: 270 mg | Fiber: 1.2 g | Carbohydrates: 7.5 g | Sugar: 4.9 g

Bean and Leek Soup

This flavorful and nutritious soup is simple, quick to prepare, and more mild-flavored than the other soups in this chapter. It goes well with a salad or can be enjoyed on its own.

INGREDIENTS | SERVES 4

2 teaspoons olive oil

4 medium leeks (bulb only), chopped

2 cloves garlic, chopped

2 cups low-sodium vegetable broth

2 (16-ounce) cans cannellini beans, drained and rinsed

2 bay leaves

2 teaspoons ground cumin

½ cup whole-wheat couscous

1. Heat olive oil in a large saucepan over medium heat. Add leeks and garlic and sauté until tender.

2. Add broth, beans, bay leaves, and cumin and bring to a boil.

3. Reduce to a simmer, stir in couscous, and simmer, covered, 5 minutes.

4. Remove bay leaves and serve warm.

Per Serving | Calories: 301 | Fat: 3.9 g | Protein: 14.72 g | Sodium: 142 mg | Fiber: 13 g | Carbohydrates: 51 g | Sugar: 5 g

Strawberry and Feta Summer Salad

This light and simple Mediterranean salad can be prepared in a matter of minutes and pairs well with any of the soups or sandwiches in this chapter.

INGREDIENTS | SERVES 2

2 cloves garlic, minced

1 teaspoon honey

1 teaspoon Dijon mustard

¼ cup raspberry vinaigrette

2 tablespoons balsamic vinegar

2 tablespoons brown sugar

1 cup olive oil

4 cups romaine lettuce

2 cups sliced strawberries

1 cup crumbled feta cheese

1. Dressing: whisk together garlic, honey, mustard, raspberry vinaigrette, balsamic vinegar, brown sugar, and olive oil until well blended.

2. Toss lettuce, strawberries, and feta cheese in a separate large bowl.

3. Divide salad between 2 serving bowls, top with dressing, and serve.

Per Serving | Calories: 304 | Fat: 17 g | Protein: 12 g | Sodium: 112 mg | Fiber: 3.8 g | Carbohydrates: 16 g | Sugar: 10 g

Baked Mozzarella Sticks

This healthy version of a popular appetizer is very easy to prepare at home and makes a great snack or side dish. Enjoy plain or serve with marinara sauce for dipping.

INGREDIENTS | MAKES 24 STICKS

12 sticks reduced-fat mozzarella string cheese, cut in half

½ cup egg whites

2 tablespoons flour

½ cup Italian bread crumbs

½ cup panko bread crumbs

2 teaspoons vegetarian Parmesan cheese

1 tablespoon dried parsley

1. Freeze mozzarella pieces at least 1 hour.

2. Place egg whites in a medium bowl and flour in a medium bowl.

3. In a third medium bowl, mix Italian bread crumbs, panko bread crumbs, Parmesan, and parsley.

4. Dip frozen mozzarella pieces in flour, roll in egg whites, then cover well with bread crumb mix.

5. Place the sticks on a baking sheet covered with parchment paper and freeze 1 hour.

6. When ready to eat, bake in a 400°F oven 10 minutes, turning halfway through.

Per Serving (1 stick) | Calories: 56 | Fat: 3.3 g | Protein: 4 g | Sodium: 113 mg | Fiber: 0.13 g | Carbohydrates: 2.4 g | Sugar: 0.3 g

Creamy Spinach Dip

This low-fat alternative to a traditional spinach dip makes a great snack and can be served with crackers, celery, or toasted bread.

INGREDIENTS | SERVES 10

1 (10-ounce) package frozen spinach, thawed and drained

½ cup light sour cream

5 tablespoons light mayonnaise

⅓ cup grated vegetarian Parmesan cheese

¼ cup chopped scallions

1 clove garlic, minced

1 cup shredded low-fat mozzarella cheese

1. Preheat oven to 375°F.

2. Combine all ingredients in a medium bowl, mixing well.

3. Transfer to a 9" × 9" glass baking dish and cook 20–25 minutes until cheese is completely melted.

Per Serving | Calories: 122 | Fat: 10 g | Protein: 5 g | Sodium: 186 mg | Fiber: 0.8 g | Carbohydrates: 2.4 g | Sugar: 0.5 g

The Multipurpose Dip

Dips are often very versatile. In addition to being delicious when served with crackers, toast, pretzels, or vegetable sticks, they can make great sandwich or salad toppings. Next time you eat a sandwich or burger, try topping it with your favorite dip to add some flavor.

Baked Ziti with Tomato and Spinach

This traditional Italian dish can be prepared with low-fat and healthy ingredient substitutions for a meal that is just as delicious reheated as it is fresh.

INGREDIENTS | SERVES 6

12 ounces uncooked ziti

3 cloves garlic, minced

1 teaspoon olive oil

1 (10-ounce) package frozen spinach, thawed and drained

1 teaspoon salt

1 teaspoon freshly ground black pepper

2 (15-ounce) cans crushed tomatoes

2 tablespoons chopped fresh basil

1 teaspoon dried oregano

2 cups shredded low-fat mozzarella, divided

¼ cup grated vegetarian Parmesan cheese

8 ounces fat-free ricotta cheese

1. Preheat oven to 375°F.

2. Prepare pasta according to package directions, stopping 3 minutes short of recommended cooking time.

3. Prepare sauce by sautéing garlic and oil in a large saucepan over medium heat 3 minutes. Add spinach, salt, pepper, tomatoes, basil, and oregano and cook 5 minutes, stirring frequently.

4. Combine sauce, pasta, half the mozzarella, Parmesan, and ricotta. Mix well and transfer to a lightly oiled 10" × 13" baking dish.

5. Top dish with remaining mozzarella and bake 30 minutes.

6. Allow to cool 5 minutes to set, then serve.

Per Serving | Calories: 372 | Fat: 11.51 g | Protein: 19 g | Sodium: 819 mg | Fiber: 3.9 g | Carbohydrates: 48 g | Sugar: 3.7 g

Butternut Squash Gratin

This spin on a traditional dish replaces the potatoes with squash for a meal with a bit more fiber and fewer total carbs. This recipe uses panko to form the traditional crusty top, but you can also add Cheddar cheese for more flavor and a bit more fat.

INGREDIENTS | SERVES 6

1 large butternut squash, peeled and thinly sliced

½ cup skim milk

2 cloves garlic, minced

⅓ cup freshly grated vegetarian Parmesan cheese, divided

¾ teaspoons salt, divided

½ teaspoon freshly ground black pepper

2 tablespoons unsalted butter, melted

½ cup panko bread crumbs

Butternut Squash: Underrated Superfood

Butternut squash is a low-fat, high-fiber, delicious food. It's excellent for overall health, and the fiber will keep you full between meals and keep your digestive system happy. It's very high in vitamin A, which is a potent fighter against breast cancer, as well as eye degeneration and the negative effects of aging.

1. Preheat oven to 400°F.

2. In a large bowl, combine squash, milk, garlic, half the Parmesan, ½ teaspoon salt, and pepper.

3. Transfer squash mixture to a lightly oiled 10" × 13" baking dish, spreading evenly.

4. In a separate small bowl, combine butter, bread crumbs, and remaining salt and Parmesan.

5. Spread bread crumb mix over the casserole and bake 30–35 minutes. Finish with an additional 2 minutes under the broiler to crisp the top.

Per Serving | Calories: 44 | Fat: 4 g | Protein: 0.8 g | Sodium: 304 mg | Fiber: 0 g | Carbohydrates: 1.4 g | Sugar: 1 g

CHAPTER 9

Seafood

Seared Chilean Sea Bass with Homemade Pesto

This light and tasty recipe uses Chilean sea bass to pack in healthy proteins and fats, but the homemade pesto can be used on any white fish for a delicious dinner.

INGREDIENTS | SERVES 4

2 cups baby spinach

½ cup fresh parsley

1 clove garlic, smashed

¼ cup chopped walnuts

2 teaspoons fresh lemon juice

¼ cup plus 1 tablespoon extra-virgin olive oil, divided

1 teaspoon salt, divided

½ teaspoon freshly ground black pepper, divided

4 (6-ounce) pieces wild-caught Chilean sea bass

1. To make the pesto, combine spinach, parsley, garlic, walnuts, lemon juice, ¼ cup oil, ½ teaspoon salt, and ¼ teaspoon pepper in a food processor and blend until smooth.

2. Heat 1 tablespoon oil in a cast iron skillet over medium-high heat.

3. When oil just begins to smoke, season sea bass lightly with remaining salt and pepper and sear 3 minutes per side.

4. Remove from skillet, top with pesto, and serve.

Per Serving | Calories: 358 | Fat: 32 g | Protein: 14.8 g | Sodium: 73.127 mg | Fiber: 1 g | Carbohydrates: 2.434 g | Sugar: 0.386 g

Wild-Caught versus Farm-Raised Fish

Whenever possible, buy wild-caught fish. It's a bit more expensive, but the quality is significantly better than farm-raised fish. Fish raised on a farm are often kept in very small confined tanks, fed low-quality food, and even fed food dye to make their meat look more appetizing. Wild-caught fish eat a natural diet and are much higher in healthy fats and nutrients.

Garlic and Herb-Roasted Salmon with Tomatoes

Of all the fish, salmon is one of the healthiest, providing good omega-3 fatty acids that act as an anti-inflammatory and improve mental functioning.

INGREDIENTS | SERVES 4

2 tablespoons extra-virgin olive oil

2 cloves garlic, minced

⅛ teaspoon cayenne pepper

1 teaspoon lemon juice

¼ cup chopped fresh parsley

1 teaspoon kosher salt

4 wild-caught salmon fillets (about 2 pounds)

12 cherry tomatoes

1 medium lemon, sliced into rounds

Choose Your Fish Wisely

When choosing fish, opt for wild-caught whenever possible. Wild-caught fish are much higher in good fats, and you can even find wild-caught fish canned and ready to eat if you don't live near an ocean or lake where fresh fish is usually plentiful.

1. Preheat oven to 450°F.

2. In a small mixing bowl, combine oil, garlic, cayenne, lemon juice, parsley, and salt, mixing well.

3. Lay the salmon skin-down on a baking sheet lined with parchment paper. Arrange cherry tomatoes and lemon slices between fillets.

4. Drizzle the fillets, lemon slices, and tomatoes with herb mixture.

5. Cook 6–8 minutes or until salmon is mostly done. Finish under the broiler 5 additional minutes to roast the lemons and tomatoes.

6. Remove and serve salmon with roasted lemon and tomatoes.

Per Serving | Calories: 388.48 | Fat: 21 g | Protein: 44.98 g | Sodium: 692 mg | Fiber: 0.622 g | Carbohydrates: 2.3 g | Sugar: 1.06 g

Crispy Parmesan Tilapia

While tilapia is low in fat, it is also a very cheap source of protein. Due to its mild flavor, it is easy to use in a variety of recipes. This crispy tilapia recipe can be served with your favorite salad or pasta.

INGREDIENTS | SERVES 4

1 cup Italian bread crumbs

¼ cup chopped fresh parsley

1 cup freshly grated Parmesan cheese

½ teaspoon salt

4 (4-ounce) tilapia fillets

¼ cup lemon juice

4 cloves garlic, minced

¼ teaspoon red pepper flakes

2 tablespoons olive oil

The Leanest Fish?

In general, white fish like cod, halibut, and tilapia are lower in fat and are a good choice when you're watching your calories. High-fat fish, like tuna or salmon, have more calories but also more good omega-3 fatty acids. The choice is yours.

1. Preheat oven to 400°F.

2. Mix bread crumbs, parsley, Parmesan, and salt in a shallow bowl or serving dish.

3. Place lemon juice in a separate shallow dish and coat tilapia in it. Next, coat fish in the bread crumb mixture before transferring to a lightly oiled baking sheet.

4. Top fillets with garlic and red pepper flakes, and drizzle or spray with olive oil to help it crisp.

5. Bake 10–12 minutes until fully cooked, then serve.

Per Serving | Calories: 185.69 | Fat: 10.2 g | Protein: 24.98 g | Sodium: 858.34 mg | Fiber: 1.49 g | Carbohydrates: 21.71 g | Sugar: 2.11 g

Clam Chowder

This hearty, traditional New England–style clam chowder is very filling and provides a good mix of protein, carbs, and fat. You can double the recipe to make a large batch to store in bulk.

INGREDIENTS | SERVES 4

1 tablespoon canola oil

1 medium celery root, peeled and chopped

2 large carrots, peeled and chopped

2 stalks celery, chopped

2 large potatoes, peeled and chopped

1 large onion, peeled and chopped

¼ teaspoon salt

¼ teaspoon freshly ground black pepper

1 (8-ounce) bottle clam juice

2 cups water

2 tablespoons cornstarch

1 cup skim milk

2 (6-ounce) cans baby clams

1 cup cooked corn kernels

1. Add oil, celery root, carrots, celery, potatoes, onion, salt, and pepper to a large stockpot. Cover and cook 12 minutes over medum heat until onions and potatoes are softened.

2. Add clam juice and water. Return to a boil over high heat, then reduce to low heat and simmer 20–25 minutes.

3. In a separate small dish, mix cornstarch and milk until starch is fully dissolved. Add mixture to soup and stir until well blended.

4. Add clams and corn. Continue to cook 5 more minutes, then serve.

Per Serving | Calories: 264.78 | Fat: 4.757 g | Protein: 7.14 g | Sodium: 364 mg | Fiber: 7.2 g | Carbohydrates: 50.93 g | Sugar: 9.941 g

Seared Tilapia with Pan Sauce

This dish sears the tilapia to crisp up the texture and lock in the flavor, and the lemon-peppercorn sauce made in the same pan is the perfect topping.

INGREDIENTS | SERVES 2

¾ cup chicken broth

¼ cup lemon juice

1½ teaspoons drained peppercorns, crushed

3 teaspoons butter, divided

1 teaspoon vegetable oil

2 (4-ounce) tilapia fillets

¼ teaspoon salt

¼ teaspoon freshly ground black pepper

¼ cup all-purpose flour

1. In a small bowl, combine broth, lemon juice, and peppercorns and set aside.

2. Add 1 teaspoon butter and oil in a large nonstick skillet over low heat.

3. Sprinkle fish fillets with salt and pepper and then dredge in flour.

4. Increase heat to medium-high, add fish to skillet, and sauté 3–4 minutes on each side.

5. Remove fish and add prepared broth mixture to pan, trying to scrape all the bits that may have stuck to the bottom of the pan. Bring liquid to a boil and then reduce heat and simmer 3–5 minutes.

6. Remove pan from heat, stir in remaining 2 teaspoons butter, pour over fillets, and serve warm.

Per Serving | Calories: 186 | Fat: 11.79 g | Protein: 24.8 g | Sodium: 1,055 mg | Fiber: 1.03 g | Carbohydrates: 19.42 g | Sugar: 0.79 g

Fish Tacos with Homemade Sauce

These delicious fish tacos with a low-fat homemade cilantro sauce are a tasty Mexican-style treat. You can make the sauce in advance to save time and keep it in the refrigerator until you're ready to use it.

INGREDIENTS | SERVES 4

¼ cup sliced green onions

¼ cup chopped cilantro

3 tablespoons fat-free mayonnaise

3 tablespoons reduced-fat sour cream

1½ teaspoons fresh lime juice

¼ teaspoon salt

1 clove garlic, minced

1 teaspoon ground cumin

1 teaspoon ground coriander

½ teaspoon smoked paprika

¼ teaspoon ground red pepper

⅛ teaspoon salt

⅛ teaspoon garlic powder

1½ pounds red snapper fillets

1 tablespoon olive oil

8 corn tortillas

2 cups shredded cabbage

Choose Your Fish

There's a wide variety of fish to choose from, all with their own unique flavors and nutritional profiles. If you're used to sticking with the basics, like tilapia and tuna, try some of the other options available at your local store. Red snapper, cod, Chilean sea bass, or any of the other fish you may find are excellent to try in this recipe.

1. Preheat oven to 425°F.

2. To make the sauce, combine green onions, cilantro, mayonnaise, sour cream, lime juice, salt, and fresh garlic in a small bowl and mix well.

3. Combine cumin, coriander, paprika, red pepper, salt, and garlic powder in a separate small bowl. Season both sides of each fillet with this mix.

4. Place seasoned fish on a lightly oiled baking sheet and cook 8–9 minutes, until fish flakes easily. Remove from oven.

5. Using a fork, break the fish into pieces to form the taco filling.

6. Heat corn tortillas according to package directions. Prepare the tacos by layering sauce, fish, and shredded cabbage in the tortillas.

Per Serving | Calories: 199.62 | Fat: 3.9 g | Protein: 35.57 g | Sodium: 342 mg | Fiber: 1.399 g | Carbohydrates: 3.8 g | Sugar: 1.5 g

Shrimp Taco Salad

If fish tacos aren't your thing, this spicy Southwestern-style Shrimp Taco Salad may be right up your alley. Packed with healthy fats, proteins, and micronutrients, this is the perfect summer dinner.

INGREDIENTS | SERVES 4

¼ cup lime juice

2 tablespoons olive oil

1 teaspoon ground cumin

2 teaspoons minced garlic

2 teaspoons chipotle hot sauce

¾ pound medium shrimp, peeled and deveined

1 cup chopped romaine lettuce

½ cup chopped green onions

¼ cup chopped cilantro

1 (15-ounce) can black beans, drained and rinsed

3 plum tomatoes, chopped

2 cups crushed tortilla chips

1. Preheat grill to medium-high.

2. Combine lime juice, oil, cumin, garlic, and hot sauce in a small bowl and set aside.

3. Place shrimp on metal grill skewers and lightly drizzle with 1 tablespoon of lime juice mixture. Grill shrimp skewers 4 minutes per side.

4. Place grilled shrimp in a large bowl and add lettuce, onions, cilantro, black beans, and tomatoes, tossing well with remaining lime mixture.

5. Evenly divide tortilla chips between 4 bowls, top with shrimp salad, and serve.

Per Serving | Calories: 247.43 | Fat: 9.09 g | Protein: 22.95 g | Sodium: 477.33 mg | Fiber: 6.22 g | Carbohydrates: 18.35 g | Sugar: 3.7 g

Bourbon Lime Salmon

Salmon is one of the best natural sources of omega-3 fatty acids, and this Asian-style recipe is easy to prepare in bulk and eat throughout the week.

INGREDIENTS | SERVES 8

1 cup packed brown sugar or brown sugar substitute

6 tablespoons bourbon

¼ cup soy sauce

2 tablespoons lime juice

2 teaspoons freshly grated ginger

½ teaspoon salt

¼ teaspoon freshly ground black pepper

2 cloves garlic, crushed

8 (6-ounce) salmon fillets

4 teaspoons sesame seeds

½ cup sliced green onions

1. Combine brown sugar, bourbon, soy sauce, lime juice, ginger, salt, pepper, and garlic in a large resealable plastic bag. Marinate salmon fillets in the bag at least 30 minutes in the refrigerator.

2. When ready to cook, preheat the broiler.

3. Transfer fish to broiler pan and discard marinade. Broil fish 10–12 minutes or until it flakes easily.

4. Sprinkle fish with sesame seeds and green onions and serve.

Per Serving | Calories: 386.41 | Fat: 11.46 g | Protein: 34.196 g | Sodium: 495.94 mg | Fiber: 0.43 g | Carbohydrates: 28.96 g | Sugar: 27.15 g

Maryland Crab Cakes

These traditional Baltimore favorites are a delicious and easy-to-prepare meal that can be enjoyed plain, served as a side dish, or made into a sandwich.

INGREDIENTS | MAKES 6 CAKES

2 slices white bread, crusts trimmed

1 pound crabmeat (available in cans at most stores)

1 large egg

1 tablespoon mayonnaise

1 teaspoon Dijon mustard

1 teaspoon Worcestershire sauce

1 tablespoon Old Bay Seasoning or other seafood seasoning

2 tablespoons butter

1. Rip bread into small pieces and add to a large bowl with crab, egg, mayonnaise, mustard, Worcestershire sauce, and Old Bay, mixing gently with a large spoon or by hand.

2. Shape mixture into 6 round patties and set aside.

3. Heat butter in a medium nonstick skillet over medium-high heat and fry cakes 3–4 minutes per side or until outsides are brown and crispy.

Per Serving (1 cake) | Calories: 137.56 | Fat: 7.44 g | Protein: 16.47 g | Sodium: 293 mg | Fiber: 0.029 g | Carbohydrates: 0.362 g | Sugar: 0.181 g

Coconut Shrimp

This low-fat version of a traditionally fried, tropical dish is easy to prepare and goes well with a fresh salad or pasta dish.

INGREDIENTS | SERVES 4

¼ cup cornstarch

1 tablespoon Caribbean jerk seasoning

2 large egg whites

1 cup sweetened flaked coconut

1 cup panko bread crumbs

1 teaspoon paprika

1½ pounds large shrimp, peeled and deveined

1. Preheat oven to 425°F.

2. Set up 3 shallow bowls. Place cornstarch and jerk seasoning in the first; egg whites in the second; and coconut, panko, and paprika in the third.

3. Dredge shrimp in the cornstarch mix, then egg whites, then panko mixture, coating shrimp on all sides.

4. Place shrimp on a wire baking rack on a baking sheet to catch any drippings.

5. Bake 10–12 minutes, turning halfway through. Remove and serve warm.

Per Serving | Calories: 218.14 | Fat: 3.01 g | Protein: 36.025 g | Sodium: 276 mg | Fiber: 0.287 g | Carbohydrates: 9.27 g | Sugar: 0.177 g

Lemon Steamed Halibut

This simple and citrusy dish works well with halibut but can also be prepared with cod, tilapia, or any other white fish instead.

INGREDIENTS | SERVES 6

6 (4-ounce) halibut fillets
1 tablespoon dried dill
1 tablespoon onion powder
2 teaspoons dried parsley
¼ teaspoon paprika
¼ teaspoon salt
¼ teaspoon lemon pepper
¼ teaspoon garlic powder
2 tablespoons lemon juice

1. Preheat oven to 375°F.

2. Cut 6 foil squares big enough to fold each fillet into its own foil packet.

3. Place a fillet on each foil square and sprinkle with dill, onion powder, parsley, paprika, salt, lemon pepper, and garlic powder, then drizzle fillets with lemon juice.

4. Fold foil around each fillet to create a sealed packet. Place packets on a large baking sheet.

5. Bake 20–25 minutes until fish flakes easily with a fork.

Per Serving | Calories: 130.58 | Fat: 2.635 g | Protein: 23.622 g | Sodium: 162 mg | Fiber: 0.35 g | Carbohydrates: 1.7 g | Sugar: 0.221 g

Grilled Tuna Teriyaki

Tuna steaks are easy to find at most stores and provide a healthy dose of protein and omega-3 fatty acids, much like salmon. This light and fresh-tasting recipe is best enjoyed soon after preparing, but it will last for a few days in the refrigerator, if necessary.

INGREDIENTS | SERVES 4

2 tablespoons soy sauce

1 tablespoon rice wine

1 tablespoon minced gingerroot

1 clove garlic, minced

4 (6-ounce) tuna steaks

1 tablespoon vegetable oil

Tuna versus Salmon

When it comes to seafood, two of the most readily available fish choices are salmon and tuna. While salmon is often considered healthier than tuna, as it is loaded with healthy fats, tuna steaks and fillets are the exception. Canned tuna may not have much nutritional benefit, but tuna steaks, particularly when wild-caught, can be just as healthy and tasty as wild-caught salmon.

1. Add soy sauce, rice wine, ginger, and garlic together in a bowl or resealable bag, stirring well. Add tuna to the marinade, turning to coat, and then marinate in the refrigerator at least 30 minutes.

2. When ready to cook, preheat a grill to medium heat, lightly coating with vegetable oil.

3. Transfer fish to grill and discard marinade. Cook tuna 3–6 minutes per side or until fully cooked through.

Per Serving | Calories: 283.44 | Fat: 11.66 g | Protein: 39.7 g | Sodium: 331 mg | Fiber: 0.11 g | Carbohydrates: 1.37 g | Sugar: 0.168 g

Spicy Grilled Shrimp Skewers

Shrimp is a mild-flavored food, but the spicy Asian sauce in this recipe brings the heat. When served warm and fresh off the grill, these skewers are the perfect pairing for a summer salad.

INGREDIENTS | SERVES 4

2 tablespoons finely chopped scallions

1 teaspoon sriracha hot sauce

1½ tablespoons Thai sweet chili sauce

2½ tablespoons light mayonnaise

40 large raw shrimp, shelled and deveined

2 teaspoons freshly ground black pepper

1. Preheat grill to medium.

2. In a small bowl, mix scallions, hot sauce, Thai sauce, and light mayonnaise, stirring well.

3. Using 8 metal skewers, place 5 shrimp on each skewer and sprinkle with pepper.

4. Grill shrimp skewers 6–8 minutes per side. Remove, coat with sauce, and serve warm.

Per Serving | Calories: 146 | Fat: 8.1 g | Protein: 14.61 g | Sodium: 239 mg | Fiber: 0.7 g | Carbohydrates: 3 g | Sugar: 0.87 g

Margarita Shrimp

These Mexican-style shrimp combine the classic flavors of tequila and lime for a refreshing and protein-packed meal.

INGREDIENTS | SERVES 4

½ tablespoon olive oil

1 pound large shrimp, peeled and deveined

¼ teaspoon ground cumin

4 cloves garlic, minced

¼ teaspoon red pepper flakes

¼ teaspoon salt

¼ teaspoon freshly ground black pepper

2 ounces tequila

2 tablespoons lime juice

1. Heat oil in a large skillet or wok over medium-high heat.

2. Season the shrimp with cumin, garlic, red pepper flakes, salt, and pepper, then add to hot oil and cook about 2 minutes per side.

3. Add tequila and cook another 30–40 seconds. Remove and drizzle with lime juice before serving.

Per Serving | Calories: 171.78 | Fat: 3.695 g | Protein: 23 g | Sodium: 314.45 mg | Fiber: 0.16 g | Carbohydrates: 2.243 g | Sugar: 0 g

Garlic and Herb Seared Salmon

If you want to give your salmon a sear and avoid a traditional baked preparation,
this recipe will give you crispy fillets with a fresh garlic flavor.

INGREDIENTS | SERVES 4

4 cloves garlic, crushed

1 teaspoon dried Herbes de Provence

1 teaspoon red wine vinegar

2 tablespoons plus 1 teaspoon olive oil, divided

2 tablespoons Dijon mustard

4 (6-ounce) wild-caught salmon fillets

4 lemon wedges for serving

1. Combine garlic, herbs, vinegar, 1 teaspoon oil, and mustard in a food processor until smooth.

2. Heat remaining 2 tablespoons of oil in a large nonstick skillet over medium-high heat and grill salmon fillets 5 minutes.

3. Flip fillets and cook 3 minutes, spooning half the garlic sauce on the cooked side of each fillet.

4. Flip fillets again, cooking 1 more minute and spreading sauce on the other side of fillets. Flip fillets one last time and cook 1 minute.

5. Remove and serve each fillet with a fresh lemon wedge.

Per Serving | Calories: 258.78 | Fat: 12.109 g | Protein: 33.87 g | Sodium: 310 mg | Fiber: 0.356 g | Carbohydrates: 1.498 g | Sugar: 0 g

Crab and Artichoke Dip

The perfect game-day appetizer, this version of a classic cheesy dip significantly lowers the fat while delivering all the flavor.

INGREDIENTS | SERVES 16

1 (14-ounce) can artichoke hearts packed in water, drained and chopped

1 pound crab meat, chopped

2 tablespoons chopped chives

6 tablespoons reduced-fat sour cream

6 tablespoons light mayonnaise

⅓ cup grated Parmesan cheese

¾ cup shredded Cheddar cheese

1 teaspoon lemon juice

1. Preheat oven to 400°F.

2. Add all ingredients to a large bowl, mixing well. Transfer mixture to a 10" × 13" glass baking dish.

3. Bake 30 minutes until top just begins to brown. Remove and serve warm.

Per Serving | Calories: 106.74 | Fat: 7.5 g | Protein: 8.3 g | Sodium: 197 mg | Fiber: 0.44 g | Carbohydrates: 1.4 g | Sugar: 0.174 g

Lower the Fat with Substitute Ingredients

With recipes that call for traditionally fatty ingredients like sour cream, mayonnaise, or cream cheese, look for low-fat options at the store. You can also substitute fat-free Greek yogurt for sour cream in most recipes. This is a very easy way to lower the calories and fat content without sacrificing all the flavor.

Beef and Poultry

Greek Chicken Quesadillas

Quesadillas are very quick to throw together, especially if you use premade ingredients. You can cook and eat them fresh or even reheat them later if you want to pack them for lunches at work or school.

INGREDIENTS | SERVES 1

2 tablespoons pesto spread

1 whole-grain tortilla

4 ounces shredded, cooked chicken

½ cup fresh baby spinach

¼ cup feta cheese

Homemade Pesto

If you have some time on your hands and really want to spice things up, homemade pesto will really set this recipe off. There are plenty of recipes out there to try, but for a simple one, take freshly chopped basil with a little minced garlic and simply mix it all up with a little olive oil. Adjust portions to taste.

1. Spread pesto all over tortilla and fill one half with chicken, spinach, and cheese.

2. Fold in half and cook in a nonstick pan over medium heat.

3. Flip once the bottom of the tortilla is golden brown. Brown the other side and serve.

Per Serving | Calories: 315 | Fat: 16 g | Protein: 38 g | Sodium: 527 mg | Fiber: 0 g | Carbohydrates: 2 g | Sugar: 2 g

Slow-Cooked Chicken

Using a slow cooker is a very easy way to cook a lot of chicken in bulk that won't result in a week's worth of dry, rubbery poultry. Throw in as many fragrant vegetables as you'd like to bump up the flavor of this chicken recipe.

INGREDIENTS | SERVES 4

1 pound boneless, skinless chicken breasts

1 (12-ounce) box low-sodium chicken broth

1 medium white onion, peeled and sliced

½ teaspoon garlic salt

½ teaspoon freshly ground black pepper

1. Place chicken in slow cooker and add enough chicken broth to cover the top of the breasts.

2. Add remaining ingredients to the slow cooker.

3. Cover and cook on low for 6 hours or until chicken is tender and shreds easily with a fork.

4. Remove, shred with a fork, and eat fresh or store for later.

Per Serving | Calories: 139 | Fat: 3 g | Protein: 24 g | Sodium: 426 mg | Fiber: 1 g | Carbohydrates: 3 g | Sugar: 1 g

The Best Way to Cook Chicken?

This might just be the best way to cook chicken. Baking and grilling are fine, but these techniques have a tendency to dry it out. By slow-cooking your chicken, it will fall apart and shred very easily and retain a lot of its moisture. The flavor by itself is good but not overpowering, so you can add it to other dishes or sauces without negatively impacting the flavor of the meal.

Southwestern Fajitas

Fajitas are a very flexible meal. Once cooked and prepared, they can be reheated and eaten alone or served with tortillas and rice for extra carbs. You can also serve these with shredded Mexican cheese and low-fat sour cream.

INGREDIENTS | SERVES 2

6 ounces boneless, skinless chicken breast, cut into strips

1 teaspoon red pepper flakes

1 teaspoon fajita or taco seasoning

1 (12-ounce) bag mixed fajita vegetables

1. Season chicken with red pepper flakes and fajita seasoning. Add to a medium nonstick skillet over medium-high heat and cook 8–10 minutes. Once cooked, remove and set aside.

2. Cook vegetables in pan and mix in chicken once vegetables are fully cooked, about 4–6 minutes.

Per Serving | Calories: 100 | Fat: 2 g | Protein: 18 g | Sodium: 195 mg | Fiber: 0 g | Carbohydrates: 0 g | Sugar: 0 g

Lemon-Herb Grilled Chicken Salad

A fresh take on grilled salad, this dish is very refreshing and perfect for the summer.

INGREDIENTS | SERVES 1

4 ounces grilled chicken breast, sliced
1 cup mixed greens
1 tablespoon olive oil
1 tablespoon lemon juice
½ teaspoon garlic salt
¼ teaspoon dried rosemary

Mix all the ingredients in a medium bowl and serve cold.

Per Serving | Calories: 251 | Fat: 16 g | Protein: 24 g | Sodium: 240 mg | Fiber: 0 g | Carbohydrates: 1 g | Sugar: 0 g

"Detox" with Lemons

While most detox diets are worthless, as your liver does a fine job cleansing you from the inside out, lemons are very beneficial and help support the detoxification process. Lemons are very alkalizing for your body, which means they help maintain a stable pH balance. They are also very good for the liver, a very important organ in the body, and lemon juice is thought to be very cleansing internally.

Pulled-Chicken BBQ Sandwiches

A very easy way to serve shredded chicken. You can use any sauce you like, including barbecue, hot wing sauce, ranch, or whatever else your favorite sauce may be.

INGREDIENTS | SERVES 1

4 ounces shredded Slow-Cooked Chicken (see recipe in this chapter)

2 tablespoons barbecue sauce (or any other sauce of your choice)

1 whole-wheat hamburger bun

Get Saucy for Maximum Flavor

Anytime you're eating precooked meat, mix up your flavor game with a variety of sauces. Barbecue sauce, hot sauce, mustard, ranch, blue cheese, ketchup...the options are endless, so there is no excuse to eat dry, boring food.

1. In a medium bowl, mix chicken and sauce until chicken is coated completely. (It's best if chicken is heated.)

2. Place chicken on sandwich bun and serve.

Per Serving | Calories: 316 | Fat: 3 g | Protein: 29 g | Sodium: 1,003 mg | Fiber: 4 g | Carbohydrates: 43 g | Sugar: 14 g

Greek Butterflied Chicken

This delicious recipe is bursting with flavor. Be sure to purchase regular chicken breasts rather than thin-sliced so they can be cut appropriately.

INGREDIENTS | SERVES 4

1 pound boneless, skinless chicken breasts

½ cup feta cheese

1 (8-ounce) package sun-dried tomatoes

2 tablespoons pesto

¼ teaspoon salt

½ teaspoon freshly ground black pepper

1. Preheat oven to 350°F.

2. Butterfly chicken breasts by slicing along the side of each breast lengthwise.

3. Lay open breasts and place cheese, tomatoes, and pesto on one side of each, then fold other side of breasts over filling mixture, using a toothpick to hold stuffed breasts shut, if necessary.

4. Season with salt and pepper and bake 35–40 minutes or until juices run clear.

Per Serving | Calories: 232 | Fat: 8 g | Protein: 29 g | Sodium: 144 mg | Fiber: 3 g | Carbohydrates: 13 g | Sugar: 9 g

Chicken and Bean Protein Burritos

Once prepared, you can slow-cook these in the oven or microwave them if you're in a hurry. You can also add low-fat sour cream or fat-free Greek yogurt if desired.

INGREDIENTS | SERVES 1

½ cup cooked pinto beans

2 teaspoons taco seasoning

2 tablespoons medium salsa

½ cup cooked rice

1 whole-wheat tortilla

3 ounces cooked chicken, shredded

2 tablespoons low-fat Mexican blend cheese

1. Blend beans, taco seasoning, and salsa in food processor.

2. Spread rice on the tortilla. Top with bean mixture and chicken. Sprinkle cheese on top.

3. Microwave 15–25 seconds or heat in the oven until cheese is melted.

Per Serving | Calories: 474 | Fat: 7 g | Protein: 32 g | Sodium: 1,202 mg | Fiber: 9 g | Carbohydrates: 72 g | Sugar: 4 g

What Rice Is the Healthiest?

It really doesn't matter what sort of rice you use. White rice, brown rice, jasmine rice, and wild rice all have very similar nutritional content. You may have heard that brown rice is healthier, but the only real difference is its speed of absorption. Brown rice absorbs slower, which is why some have issues digesting it, so it's really personal preference.

Lemon-Herb Chicken

Simple to make, delicious, and stores well if you want to cook it in bulk. The seasonings add a lot of flavor with minimal extra calories, so if you want some lean and tasty protein in your diet, this recipe is for you.

INGREDIENTS | SERVES 4

⅓ cup lemon juice

⅓ cup Dijon mustard

1 tablespoon dried sage

1 tablespoon dried thyme

3 cloves garlic, crushed

4 (4-ounce) boneless, skinless, chicken breasts

Cooking spray

2 scallions, sliced

1. In a small bowl, mix together lemon juice, mustard, sage, thyme, and garlic.

2. Put chicken breasts on a plate. Coat both sides with half the lemon juice mixture and set aside 10 minutes.

3. Coat a large skillet with cooking spray and cook chicken breasts 5 minutes on each side. Use the other half of the lemon juice mixture to coat chicken as it cooks.

4. Scatter scallions over chicken before serving.

Per Serving | Calories: 155 | Fat: 4 g | Protein: 25 g | Sodium: 372 mg | Fiber: 1 g | Carbohydrates: 4 g | Sugar: 1 g

Tuscan-Style Slow Cooker Chicken

*This is another delicious slow cooker recipe that adds a
bit more flavor than the usual slow-cooked recipe.*

INGREDIENTS | SERVES 4

¼ cup chopped onion

½ medium red bell pepper, seeded and
cut into strips

½ medium green bell pepper, seeded
and cut into strips

8 ounces black beans, drained and
rinsed

4 (4-ounce) boneless, skinless chicken
breasts

2 tablespoons olive oil

1 large tomato, diced

¼ cup low-sodium chicken broth

1 tablespoon apple cider vinegar

½ teaspoon dried oregano

1 clove garlic, crushed

¼ teaspoon salt

1. Put onion, peppers, and beans in a slow cooker.

2. Place chicken on top of vegetables and beans.

3. In a bowl, stir together oil, tomato, broth, vinegar, oregano, garlic, and salt. Pour mixture over chicken.

4. Cook on low 6–7 hours and then serve.

Per Serving | Calories: 256 | Fat: 10 g | Protein: 28 g | Sodium:
179 mg | Fiber: 4 g | Carbohydrates: 13 g | Sugar: 4 g

Beer Can Chicken

This classic barbecue recipe uses beer to add a lot of moisture to your chicken from the inside. It'll be dripping with juices when you cut it open. You can also prepare the recipe with a can of Coke if you don't want to use alcohol.

INGREDIENTS | SERVES 4

1 (3–5-pound) whole medium chicken

2 tablespoons olive oil or other vegetable oil

1 tablespoon kosher salt

1 tablespoon freshly ground black pepper

2 tablespoons chopped fresh thyme leaves or 1 tablespoon dried thyme

1 (12-ounce) can beer, room temperature

1. Prepare grill for indirect heat cooking by turning on only one side of burners to medium-high and allowing entire grill to heat to 350°F.

2. Remove innards from chicken and discard. Brush chicken lightly with oil.

3. In a small bowl, combine salt, pepper, and thyme and cover chicken with rub mixture.

4. Open beer, pour out half, and use a knife to carefully cut openings into the top half of the open can. Carefully stand the chicken upright, so that the can is inside its cavity, and place the entire chicken on the cool side of the grill, making sure it stands up on its own.

5. Do not open the grill for at least 1 hour, then check every 15 minutes until fully cooked. A thermometer inserted should read 160–165°F when fully cooked.

6. Remove, allow to rest at least 10 minutes, then cut and serve.

Per Serving | Calories: 368 | Fat: 14 g | Protein: 49 g | Sodium: 144 mg | Fiber: 1 g | Carbohydrates: 4 g | Sugar: 0 g

Gameday Chicken Power Nachos

This delicious and protein-packed snack is a great way to satisfy cravings and get a well-rounded meal containing protein, carbs, and fat.

INGREDIENTS | SERVES 1

1 serving whole-grain tortilla chips

3 ounces cooked, shredded chicken

¼ cup low-fat shredded Mexican blend cheese

2 cups salsa

¼ cup low-fat sour cream

1. Spread chips on microwavable plate or bowl.

2. Top with chicken and cheese. Heat 2 minutes or until cheese is melted.

3. Remove plate from microwave and top with salsa and sour cream.

Per Serving | Calories: 522 | Fat: 20 g | Protein: 37 g | Sodium: 3,488 mg | Fiber: 10 g | Carbohydrates: 56 g | Sugar: 20 g

Baked Chicken Fingers

This recipe is sure to please the whole family and is very simple to prepare.

INGREDIENTS | SERVES 6

1½ cups buttermilk

2 teaspoons salt

1 teaspoon freshly ground black pepper

2 teaspoons paprika

1 pound boneless, skinless chicken breasts, cut into strips

1½ cups Italian bread crumbs

1. Combine buttermilk, salt, pepper, and paprika in a large resealable plastic bag. Add chicken and allow it to marinate in the refrigerator at least 6 hours.

2. Preheat oven to 450°F.

3. When ready to cook, remove chicken and discard marinade. Roll chicken in bread crumbs on a shallow plate to coat. Place chicken on a baking sheet lined with parchment paper.

4. Bake 15 minutes or until chicken strips are golden brown.

Per Serving | Calories: 204 | Fat: 2 g | Protein: 21 g | Sodium: 1,380 mg | Fiber: 1 g | Carbohydrates: 23 g | Sugar: 4 g

Salsa Verde Chicken

This Southwestern-style chicken is low in fat and high in flavor.
Try using different types of salsa to experiment with different flavors.

INGREDIENTS | SERVES 4

1 pound boneless, skinless chicken breasts

1 tablespoon olive oil

1 teaspoon garlic salt

1 (16-ounce) jar salsa verde

1½ cups shredded low-fat Monterey jack cheese

¼ cup chopped cilantro

1 medium lime, cut into wedges

1. Preheat oven to 400°F.

2. In 10" × 13" baking dish, arrange chicken breasts. Brush them with oil and season with garlic salt. Pour salsa over chicken, spreading it evenly all over.

3. Bake 30–35 minutes until chicken is fully cooked. Remove from oven, top with cheese, and finish under the broiler 1–2 minutes to melt the cheese.

4. Garnish with cilantro and lime wedges and serve.

Per Serving | Calories: 393 | Fat: 19 g | Protein: 46 g | Sodium: 2,105 mg | Fiber: 0 g | Carbohydrates: 12 g | Sugar: 0 g

Southwestern Chicken

This chicken goes well with anything. Serve it hot over white rice and fajita vegetables or enjoy it cold, sliced, and served with a salad and avocado.

INGREDIENTS | SERVES 4

½ cup olive oil, divided

¼ cup lime juice

¼ teaspoon red pepper flakes

1 tablespoon honey

½ teaspoon cumin

2 (6-ounce) boneless, skinless chicken breasts

1. In a small bowl, combine ¼ cup oil, lime juice, red pepper flakes, honey, and cumin and mix well.

2. Place chicken in a medium bowl or dish and pour the dressing on top. Cover and marinate at least 1 hour in the refrigerator.

3. When ready to cook, heat a grill or skillet to medium-high, brush grill with remaining oil using a paper towel and grilling tongs, and cook chicken 6–8 minutes per side or until fully cooked.

Per Serving | Calories: 322 | Fat: 29 g | Protein: 12 g | Sodium: 44 mg | Fiber: 0 g | Carbohydrates: 4 g | Sugar: 4 g

Spicy Avocado Turkey Burger

*This recipe kicks up the intensity of your traditional turkey burger with
the addition of sriracha, everyone's favorite hot sauce.*

INGREDIENTS | SERVES 4

4 turkey burger patties

1 teaspoon salt

1 teaspoon freshly ground black pepper

4 slices pepper jack cheese

2 medium avocados, diced

½ medium onion, peeled and chopped

2 cloves garlic, pressed

3 tablespoons lime juice

3 tablespoons sriracha or other hot sauce

1. Season burgers with salt and pepper and cook on a preheated grill or grill pan over high heat 5–6 minutes per side or until fully cooked. Add cheese to burgers and cover during last minute of cook time to melt.

2. In a medium bowl, mash together avocado, onion, garlic, and lime juice, mixing until smooth.

3. Top each burger with avocado spread and sriracha and serve.

Per Serving | Calories: 348 | Fat: 25 g | Protein: 25 g | Sodium: 342 mg | Fiber: 5 g | Carbohydrates: 8 g | Sugar: 1 g

Argentinian-Style Grilled Sirloin

A delicious twist on a traditional sirloin, this minimalist recipe allows the flavor of the steak to come through while providing a mild kick from the fresh seasonings.

INGREDIENTS | SERVES 2

2 tablespoons water

½ cup chopped fresh parsley leaves

½ cup chopped fresh cilantro leaves

1 tablespoon lemon juice

1 tablespoon olive oil

¼ teaspoon salt

¼ teaspoon freshly ground black pepper

½ teaspoon red pepper flakes

2 (4-ounce) sirloin steaks

1. In a medium bowl, combine water, parsley, cilantro, lemon juice, oil, salt, black pepper, and pepper flakes. Mix well.

2. Place steak on grill rack or skillet over medium-high heat and cook about 4 minutes per side.

3. Transfer steak to cutting board and let stand 10 minutes. Thinly slice steaks across the grain. Top with parsley and cilantro mixture before serving.

Per Serving | Calories: 222 | Fat: 13 g | Protein: 24 g | Sodium: 365 mg | Fiber: 1 g | Carbohydrates: 2 g | Sugar: 0 g

Skinny Meatballs

This recipe calls for the leanest beef you can find to minimize the fat. If you want more fat, you can use beef with a higher fat ratio, or if you want to stay low-fat but use a different meat, you can substitute the beef for ground turkey, bison, or chicken.

INGREDIENTS | SERVES 5

1 pound extra lean ground beef
½ cup minced onion
2 large egg whites
1 large egg
¼ cup oat bran
2 tablespoons low-fat Parmesan cheese
1 teaspoon oregano
½ teaspoon garlic powder
2 tablespoons skim milk
¼ teaspoon salt
¼ teaspoon freshly ground black pepper
2 tablespoons olive oil

1. Preheat oven to 375°F.

2. In a large bowl, mix all ingredients together.

3. Shape mixture into 20 balls.

4. Lay on a lightly oiled 10" × 13" baking pan and bake 30–35 minutes, turning halfway through to ensure even browning.

Per Serving | Calories: 201 | Fat: 10 g | Protein: 22 g | Sodium: 214 mg | Fiber: 1 g | Carbohydrates: 5 g | Sugar: 1 g

Steakhouse Blue Cheese Burger

This delicious burger combines the rich taste of beef with the sharp kick of blue cheese, reminiscent of a blue-cheese crusted filet mignon. Serve on a burger or with a fresh side salad.

INGREDIENTS | SERVES 4

1 pound lean ground beef

1 large egg

¼ cup bread crumbs

1 tablespoon steak seasoning

½ cup blue cheese crumbles

1. In a large bowl, combine beef, egg, bread crumbs, and seasoning. Form mixture into 4 evenly shaped patties.

2. Start to cook patties over a grill or medium skillet preheated to medium-high heat. Cook for about 3–4 minutes on the first side then flip; sprinkle blue cheese crumbles on top of the patties and allow to melt as it cooks to your desired level of doneness.

Per Serving | Calories: 301 | Fat: 18 g | Protein: 28 g | Sodium: 376 mg | Fiber: 0 g | Carbohydrates: 5 g | Sugar: 1 g

Hearty Beef Stew

Prep time is quick for this stew, and you can add everything to the slow cooker before you leave for work, ensuring you'll come home to a tender, fresh dinner.

INGREDIENTS | SERVES 4

4 medium red potatoes, cut into quarters

⅓ cup flour

½ teaspoon salt

¼ teaspoon freshly ground black pepper

1 pound beef stew meat

1 (14-ounce) can diced tomatoes, with liquid

2 cups water

3 cups frozen stir-fry vegetables

1. Add potatoes, flour, salt, pepper, beef, tomatoes, and water to slow cooker and mix well.

2. Cook on low 7–8 hours, until beef and potatoes are tender.

3. Add frozen stir-fry vegetables, cook another 30 minutes, and serve.

Per Serving | Calories: 281 | Fat: 8 g | Protein: 27 g | Sodium: 362 mg | Fiber: 3 g | Carbohydrates: 24 g | Sugar: 3 g

Swedish-Style Meatballs

These homemade meatballs are much healthier than the frozen meatballs you can buy at the store. To serve in traditional Swedish fashion, serve with gravy and lingonberry jam.

INGREDIENTS | MAKES 20 MEATBALLS

1 teaspoon olive oil
1 small onion, peeled and minced
1 clove garlic, minced
1 stalk celery, minced
¼ cup minced parsley
1 pound lean ground beef
1 large egg
¼ cup bread crumbs
½ teaspoon salt
¼ teaspoon freshly ground black pepper
½ teaspoon allspice
2 cups beef stock

1. Heat oil in a large skillet over medium heat and sauté onions and garlic 5 minutes.

2. Add celery and parsley and cook 3 more minutes or until celery softens, then set aside.

3. In a large bowl, combine beef, egg, onion mixture, bread crumbs, salt, pepper, and allspice, mixing well. Form into roughly 20 balls, using about 2 tablespoons of meat mixture for each.

4. Add beef stock to the pan that the celery cooked in and bring to a boil. Add meatballs, cover, and cook 20 minutes, stirring occasionally.

5. Serve warm.

Per Serving (1 meatball) | Calories: 56 | Fat: 3 g | Protein: 6 g | Sodium: 79 mg | Fiber: 0 g | Carbohydrates: 2 g | Sugar: 0 g

Balsamic Grilled Steak

This healthy and tasty steak recipe is super tender because of its special marinade and goes well with a fresh salad or rice.

INGREDIENTS | SERVES 6

1 teaspoon kosher salt

¼ cup balsamic vinegar

1 tablespoon olive oil

1 clove garlic, minced

1 tablespoon rosemary

1½ pounds flank steak

Clean Your Equipment

Food safety is a crucial part of staying healthy, and a big part of this is keeping your grill clean between uses. Just because you're cooking over a hot fire, doesn't mean you're necessarily killing any bacteria left on the grill. To keep your food safe, thoroughly brush your grill grates clean with a grill cleaning brush after each use.

1. In a large resealable plastic bag or covered dish, combine salt, vinegar, oil, garlic, and rosemary. Add steak and allow to marinate overnight.

2. When ready to cook, heat a grill to high, lightly oil the grates, and cook to desired doneness.

Per Serving | Calories: 240 | Fat: 13 g | Protein: 25 g | Sodium: 304 mg | Fiber: 1 g | Carbohydrates: 5 g | Sugar: 3 g

Beef and Broccoli Kebabs

These kabobs are full of healthy fats and nutrients from the broccoli and are quick and easy to throw on the grill for those summer parties.

INGREDIENTS | SERVES 4

⅓ cup soy sauce

¼ cup brown sugar substitute

2 tablespoons lime juice

1 tablespoon ground ginger

1 pound lean sirloin steak, cut into cubes

2 cups whole broccoli florets

2 tablespoons olive oil

3 tablespoons freshly ground black pepper

1. In a large bowl, mix soy sauce, sugar substitute, lime juice, and ginger. Add steak and toss until coated. Cover bowl and marinate in the refrigerator at least 30 minutes.

2. When ready to cook, toss broccoli in olive oil, remove steak from marinade, and place meat and vegetables on 8 metal grilling skewers. Season with pepper.

3. Grill over medium-high heat until cooked to desired doneness, about 6–8 minutes for medium-rare, longer if you want a higher cook temperature, and serve.

Per Serving | Calories: 256 | Fat: 13 g | Protein: 27 g | Sodium: 791 mg | Fiber: 3 g | Carbohydrates: 9 g | Sugar: 1 g

Orange-Flavored Beef Stir-Fry

This low-fat spin on a classic Chinese dish is a healthy alternative that's easy to prepare at home. This is a mild recipe; for extra spice, try adding some hot sauce or chili peppers.

INGREDIENTS | SERVES 4

2 medium oranges, whole

2 cloves garlic, minced

2 tablespoons soy sauce

1 tablespoon cornstarch

1 tablespoon cold water

1½ pounds sirloin, cut into thin strips

2 medium oranges, peeled and sliced

3 green onions, sliced

1 tablespoon sesame seeds

Save Time with Stir-Fry Mixes

If you enjoy making stir-fry dishes, check your frozen vegetable section for premade stir-fry mixes. You can often find frozen packages of assorted vegetables that are ready to throw in the pan with your protein of choice for a quick and healthy meal.

1. In a small bowl, grate zest from 1 orange and squeeze juice from 2 oranges. Add garlic and soy sauce and stir.

2. In a separate small bowl, mix cornstarch with cold water and add to orange juice bowl.

3. In a large skillet over medium heat, cook beef strips until browned on all sides and cooked to desired doneness, roughly 6–8 minutes.

4. Set beef aside and pour juice mix into skillet, boiling until juice thickens. Return beef to skillet and add orange segments, green onion, and sesame seeds, tossing well before serving.

Per Serving | Calories: 373 | Fat: 13 g | Protein: 38 g | Sodium: 365 mg | Fiber: 5 g | Carbohydrates: 25 g | Sugar: 17 g

Sirloin Chopped Salad

A delicious, low-carb salad option, it's a little more interesting than your standard grilled chicken salad and contains a variety of healthy fats to keep you full. Cook sirloin or your favorite cut of steak in advance, and you'll have healthy protein ready to go whenever you need it.

INGREDIENTS | SERVES 1

2 cups mixed greens

4 ounces cooked sirloin, cut into strips

¼ cup blue cheese crumbles

¼ cup balsamic vinaigrette or dressing of choice

Add greens and sirloin to a large bowl and toss well. Top with blue cheese and drizzle with balsamic dressing before serving.

Per Serving | Calories: 405 | Fat: 29 g | Protein: 31 g | Sodium: 540 mg | Fiber: 0 g | Carbohydrates: 4 g | Sugar: 3 g

What Steak to Use?

Steaks will vary cut to cut, so there is no clear-cut best steak option. If you want lower fat, generally sirloin will be a good choice. If you prefer a little more fat and flavor, rib eye is a good option.

CHAPTER 11

Pasta

Quick Ramen with Shredded Chicken

This recipe is very quick to put together and a good way to use premade chicken. All you need is chicken, a package of ramen, and a few side ingredients to make this delicious dish.

INGREDIENTS | SERVES 4

3 cups water

1 (3-ounce) package chicken-flavored ramen noodles, with seasoning package

2 cups cooked, shredded chicken breast

2 bok choy leaves, sliced into strips

1 medium carrot, sliced and peeled

1 teaspoon sesame oil

1. Bring water to a boil in a large pot.

2. Add all other ingredients and simmer 3–5 minutes before serving.

Per Serving | Calories: 225 | Fat: 7 g | Protein: 24 g | Sodium: 476 mg | Fiber: 1 g | Carbohydrates: 14 g | Sugar: 1 g

Ramen: The Cheapest Carbohydrate

Ramen may take you back to your college days, and yes, it's processed and full of sodium. However, when on a budget, ramen is very cheap, easy to prepare, and comes in all sorts of flavors. If you make it fit your macros, it's perfectly fine to enjoy some cheap ramen from time to time.

Spicy Buffalo Macaroni and Cheese

This recipe combines two classic American flavors—buffalo chicken and macaroni and cheese. It contains significantly less fat than you'd get at restaurants that serve mac and cheese, so you can enjoy this dish guilt-free.

INGREDIENTS | SERVES 2

2 cups macaroni

1 tablespoon butter

½ cup fat-free shredded Cheddar cheese

6 ounces grilled chicken, cut into strips

2 tablespoons Frank's RedHot Original Cayenne Pepper Sauce

½ cup blue cheese crumbles

1. Cook pasta according to package directions, drain, and return to pot.

2. Stir in butter and Cheddar cheese until cheese begins to melt.

3. Top with grilled chicken, drizzle with hot sauce, add blue cheese, and serve.

Per Serving | Calories: 750 | Fat: 25 g | Protein: 48 g | Sodium: 612 mg | Fiber: 4 g | Carbohydrates: 81 g | Sugar: 3 g

High-Protein Spaghetti

This incredibly simple recipe is packed with protein and carbs with minimal fat. It calls for lean ground turkey, which can quickly be prepared in bulk ahead of time to add protein to your favorite meals.

INGREDIENTS | SERVES 2

2 cups dry whole-wheat spaghetti

8 ounces ground turkey, browned

1 cup spaghetti sauce

2 tablespoons grated Parmesan cheese

1. Cook pasta according to package directions and drain.

2. Add turkey and sauce to pasta, mixing well.

3. Sprinkle with grated Parmesan and serve.

Per Serving | Calories: 601 | Fat: 14 g | Protein: 39 g | Sodium: 758 mg | Fiber: 12 g | Carbohydrates: 87 g | Sugar: 8 g

Ground Turkey—Protein on Standby

It can be hard to reach your protein goal, especially if you have to cook fresh protein every time you eat. A useful trick is to simply cook a lot of ground turkey in a pan with minimal seasoning. You can store this and add it to pasta, eggs, burritos, or any other dish that needs a protein boost. It's a very versatile addition that doesn't have an overpowering flavor.

Traditional Shrimp Scampi

Shrimp scampi is a delicious meal that is made using simple ingredients. This recipe uses orzo, but you can substitute your favorite pasta, if desired, or serve plain over steamed vegetables to reduce the carbohydrate count in this recipe.

INGREDIENTS | SERVES 4

1 cup dry orzo

½ teaspoon salt

2 tablespoons chopped parsley

4 tablespoons butter, divided

1½ pounds jumbo shrimp, peeled and deveined

1 clove garlic, minced

1. Cook orzo according to package directions. Stir in salt and parsley and set aside.

2. In a medium skillet, heat 2 tablespoons butter over medium-high heat. Sauté shrimp 2–3 minutes or until nearly cooked through and then set aside.

3. Combine remaining 2 tablespoons butter and garlic in pan and cook 30 seconds before returning shrimp to the pan.

4. Mix shrimp and garlic butter well and serve with orzo.

Per Serving | Calories: 249 | Fat: 13 g | Protein: 12 g | Sodium: 614 mg | Fiber: 1 g | Carbohydrates: 22 g | Sugar: 1 g

Mediterranean Shrimp Penne

This garlicky shrimp and pasta dish provides healthy carbohydrates and protein while minimizing the fat content traditionally found in dishes like shrimp scampi.

INGREDIENTS | SERVES 4

1 (16-ounce) package whole-grain penne
2 tablespoons olive oil
¼ cup chopped red onion
1 tablespoon chopped garlic
¼ cup white wine
2 (12-ounce) cans diced tomatoes
1 pound shrimp, peeled and deveined
1 cup grated Parmesan cheese

1. Cook pasta according to package directions and set aside.

2. Heat oil in a medium nonstick skillet over medium-high heat. Add onion and garlic, cooking about 5 minutes until onion becomes tender.

3. Add wine and tomatoes and cook 10 more minutes, stirring frequently.

4. Add shrimp to sauce and cook an additional 5 minutes. Toss shrimp with pasta and serve with Parmesan sprinkled on top.

Per Serving | Calories: 658 | Fat: 18 g | Protein: 37 g | Sodium: 1,196 mg | Fiber: 12 g | Carbohydrates: 90 g | Sugar: 7 g

Tuna Pasta Salad with Feta

This recipe packs protein, healthy fats, and healthy whole-grain pasta.

INGREDIENTS | SERVES 2

1 cup whole-grain dry macaroni

1 (5-ounce) can tuna, drained and rinsed

⅓ cup feta cheese

3 cherry tomatoes

1 tablespoon olive oil

¼ teaspoon salt

¼ teaspoon freshly ground black pepper

1. Cook pasta according to package directions and drain.

2. Add tuna and feta cheese to hot pasta, stirring until cheese begins to melt.

3. Add remaining ingredients, mix well, and serve.

Per Serving | Calories: 467 | Fat: 20 g | Protein: 32 g | Sodium: 816 mg | Fiber: 5.5 g | Carbohydrates: 43 g | Sugar: 3 g

Whole-Grain versus Regular Pasta

In terms of total calories, there really isn't too much of a difference between whole-grain and regular pastas. However, many whole-grain pastas are higher in fiber and protein, so that alone is enough reason to use them if you can find a good brand of whole-grain pasta at your local store.

Chicken and Pesto Farfalle

This is a low-fat and high-protein dish with minimal ingredients for an easy preparation.

INGREDIENTS | SERVES 2

8 ounces dry farfalle

½ cup reserved pasta water

½ pound fresh green beans, ends trimmed

½ cup reduced-fat pesto sauce

2 cups grilled chicken, cut into bite-sized pieces

1. Cook pasta according to package directions and drain, reserving ½ cup pasta water.

2. Place green beans in a shallow 8" pan with enough fresh water to cover them. Steam beans over medium heat 15 minutes and drain.

3. Combine pasta, pesto, reserved water, chicken, and green beans in a large bowl and stir to combine. This dish can be served hot or refrigerated for later and served chilled.

Per Serving | Calories: 792 | Fat: 20 g | Protein: 48 g | Sodium: 515 mg | Fiber: 7 g | Carbohydrates: 99 g | Sugar: 12 g

Orzo and Shrimp Salad

This unique spin on a pasta salad uses orzo, shrimp, and Mediterranean flavors.

INGREDIENTS | SERVES 4

8 ounces dry orzo
1 pound cooked shrimp, tails removed
1 cup cherry tomatoes, sliced in half
2 ounces reduced-fat feta cheese
¼ cup chopped basil
1 tablespoon olive oil
1 tablespoon lemon juice
1 teaspoon salt
1 teaspoon freshly ground black pepper

1. Cook pasta according to package directions. Drain and rinse under cool water.

2. Combine orzo with shrimp, tomatoes, feta cheese, basil, olive oil, and lemon juice in a large bowl.

3. Season with salt and pepper, mix well, and serve.

Per Serving | Calories: 420 | Fat: 9 g | Protein: 34 g | Sodium: 1,733 mg | Fiber: 3 g | Carbohydrates: 45 g | Sugar: 4 g

Salmon and Spinach Fettuccine

This dish is packed with omega-3 fatty acids from the salmon and healthy nutrients from the spinach.

INGREDIENTS | SERVES 2

8 ounces dry fettuccine
¼ cup butter
1 cup fat-free milk
1 tablespoon flour or flour substitute
1 cup freshly grated Parmesan cheese
½ pound smoked salmon, chopped
1 cup chopped fresh spinach
2 tablespoons capers
¼ cup chopped sun-dried tomatoes
½ cup chopped fresh oregano

1. Bring a large pot of lightly salted water to a boil. Add fettuccine and cook 11–13 minutes.

2. In a medium saucepan over medium heat, melt butter and stir in milk.

3. Mix in flour to thicken. Gradually stir in Parmesan until melted.

4. Crumble salmon into sauce. Stir in spinach, capers, sun-dried tomatoes, and oregano. Cook and stir about 3 minutes and serve over fettuccine.

Per Serving | Calories: 1,048 | Fat: 45 g | Protein: 61 g | Sodium: 1,815 mg | Fiber: 5 g | Carbohydrates: 99 g | Sugar: 12 g

Light Fettuccine Alfredo

Fettuccine Alfredo is one of the heaviest, fattiest, cream-based pasta dishes around...at least it was, before this low-fat version.

INGREDIENTS | SERVES 2

12 ounces dry fettuccine

2½ teaspoons salt, divided

1 head broccoli, cut into florets, stalk peeled and sliced

1½ cups skim milk

1 tablespoon unsalted butter

1 tablespoon flour

¾ cup freshly grated Parmesan cheese, plus more for serving

1. Cook pasta according to package directions. Drain.

2. Bring a pot of water with 1 teaspoon salt to a boil and cook broccoli 3 minutes until tender.

3. Heat milk and butter in a large saucepan over low heat and slowly whisk in flour until thickened.

4. Remove from heat and stir in Parmesan and remaining salt. Add pasta and broccoli and cook, stirring over low heat until heated through, about 3–5 minutes.

Per Serving | Calories: 958 | Fat: 21 g | Protein: 46 g | Sodium: 1,278 mg | Fiber: 8 g | Carbohydrates: 144 g | Sugar: 16 g

Lemon, Herb, and Cheese Pasta

This light and refreshing pasta pairs perfectly with chicken, shrimp, or a side salad.

INGREDIENTS | SERVES 4

1 (16-ounce) package penne
½ cup reserved pasta water
2 tablespoons butter
1 cup ricotta cheese
Zest of 1 medium lemon
¾ teaspoon salt
¼ teaspoon freshly ground black pepper

1. Cook pasta according to package directions and drain, reserving ½ cup pasta water. Return pasta to the pot.

2. In a medium bowl, whisk together pasta water, butter, and ricotta until a rich, creamy sauce forms.

3. Pour sauce over hot pasta. Add zest, salt, and pepper and toss.

Per Serving | Calories: 579 | Fat: 16 g | Protein: 22 g | Sodium: 496 mg | Fiber: 4 g | Carbohydrates: 87 g | Sugar: 4 g

Asian Shrimp Noodles

This recipe provides protein, fiber, and a delicious Asian-inspired flavor to top it all off.

INGREDIENTS | SERVES 2

1 (16-ounce) package dry rice noodles

1 bunch green onions

1 tablespoon finely chopped fresh ginger

3 tablespoons olive oil

1 pound shrimp, peeled and deveined

1 teaspoon salt

1 teaspoon freshly ground black pepper

¾ cup water

⅓ cup soy sauce

2 (12-ounce) bags shredded cabbage mix for coleslaw

1. Cook noodles according to package directions and drain, rinsing under cold water.

2. In a large skillet over medium heat, sauté green onions and ginger with olive oil 2 minutes.

3. Add shrimp to skillet in single layer with salt and pepper. Cook 3–4 minutes or until shrimp just turn opaque, stirring frequently. Remove shrimp and set aside.

4. Add water and soy sauce to the same skillet, scraping up browned bits. Stir in cabbage mix and cover and cook 6 minutes over medium heat, stirring often.

5. Transfer cabbage and shrimp mix to a bowl with noodles, mixing well before serving.

Per Serving | Calories: 1,193 | Fat: 24 g | Protein: 48 g | Sodium: 5,192 mg | Fiber: 5 g | Carbohydrates: 187 g | Sugar: 2 g

Garlic Buttered Pasta

This is the simplest yet most delicious comfort food. It can be enjoyed plain as a side dish or topped with shrimp for a lean meal.

INGREDIENTS | SERVES 2

2 cups dry angel hair pasta, or other pasta of choice

1 tablespoon butter

2 tablespoons shredded Parmesan cheese

1 clove garlic, minced

Pinch dried parsley

1. Cook pasta according to package directions and drain.

2. Mix pasta with butter, cheese, and garlic and top with parsley before serving.

Per Serving | Calories: 500 | Fat: 9 g | Protein: 18 g | Sodium: 110 mg | Fiber: 4 g | Carbohydrates: 85 g | Sugar: 3 g

CHAPTER 12

Soups and Side Dishes

Corn and Bacon Chowder

A filling, higher-fat soup, this recipe is perfect for low-carb days on your plan.

INGREDIENTS | SERVES 4

½ cup chopped celery

½ cup chopped onion

2 (16-ounce) packages frozen corn, thawed and divided

2 cups skim milk, divided

½ teaspoon salt

¼ teaspoon freshly ground black pepper

¾ cup fat-free shredded Cheddar cheese

2 slices bacon, cooked and crumbled

1. Sauté celery, onion, and 1 package corn in a stockpot over medium heat 5 minutes or until tender.

2. In a blender, blend the remaining package corn and 1 cup skim milk until smooth.

3. Add blended corn and milk mixture to pan with vegetables. Add remaining milk, salt, pepper, and cheese.

4. Cook, stirring constantly, until cheese melts. Serve topped with crumbled bacon bits.

Per Serving | Calories: 347 | Fat: 9 g | Protein: 20 g | Sodium: 612 mg | Fiber: 7 g | Carbohydrates: 56 g | Sugar: 28 g

Crumbled Bacon for Maximum Flavor

One way to add amazing flavor to your favorite dishes is by sprinkling on some crumbled bacon bits instead of using traditional salt. You need to be careful, as this does increase the fat content, but it's a lot tastier and a lot more fun than sticking with regular salt. Cook 4–6 slices until crispy, allow to cool, crumble into a resealable plastic bag or airtight container, and store until ready to use.

Sweet Potato Soup

Sweet potatoes form the base of this delicious soup, and they are one of the healthiest starchy carb sources you can eat, containing fiber and many rich nutrients.

INGREDIENTS | SERVES 4

6 large sweet potatoes, peeled and chopped

1 large onion, peeled and chopped

3 stalks celery, chopped

2 teaspoons poultry seasoning

1 quart chicken stock

2 cups skim milk

What's the Best Potato?

All potatoes are very good for you and are easy-to-prepare carb sources, but dark-colored potatoes tend to be richer in vitamins and minerals. Sweet potatoes are full of fiber, vitamin C, and beta-carotene, making them both delicious and very healthy. If you want to mix things up, another healthy potato is the Japanese potato, or purple potato, which has a rich, nutty flavor.

1. Add sweet potatoes, onion, celery, and poultry seasoning to a large pot.

2. Add chicken stock and top off with water until vegetables are just covered.

3. Boil until vegetables are soft and tender.

4. Transfer vegetables to a blender, blend softened vegetables until smooth, add milk, and return to pot to heat to desired temperature before serving.

Per Serving | Calories: 262 | Fat: 3 g | Protein: 10 g | Sodium: 390 mg | Fiber: 6 g | Carbohydrates: 49 g | Sugar: 16 g

Garlic Cheddar Cauliflower Soup

This is a cheesy, delicious, and healthy soup that's sure to please everyone, even those who don't like cauliflower, as the seasonings provide a nice flavor.

INGREDIENTS | SERVES 2

2 tablespoons olive oil

1 small yellow onion, peeled and chopped

2 cloves garlic, minced

1 medium cauliflower head, rinsed and chopped

4 cups low-sodium chicken broth

½ cup grated Parmesan cheese

1. Heat olive oil in a large saucepan over medium heat and add onion and garlic.

2. After 5 minutes, add cauliflower and chicken stock, bringing to a boil.

3. Reduce heat and simmer 20 minutes or until cauliflower is soft.

4. Transfer mixture to a blender and blend in batches until smooth.

5. Return to pan, stir in Parmesan, and heat through before serving.

Per Serving | Calories: 341 | Fat: 21 g | Protein: 17 g | Sodium: 670 mg | Fiber: 6 g | Carbohydrates: 24 g | Sugar: 7 g

Garlic Mashed Sweet Potatoes

This recipe takes a bit longer to prepare, but the garlic provides a delicious spin on traditional mashed potatoes.

INGREDIENTS | SERVES 5

4 sweet potatoes, peeled and cubed
1 teaspoon salt
1 tablespoon butter
3 cloves garlic, crushed
½ cup skim milk
2 tablespoons light sour cream

Boost Your Health with Garlic

In addition to being very tasty, garlic packs a lot of nutrients and is very good for boosting your immune system. If you find yourself coming down with a cold or feeling a bit under the weather for any other reason, try some garlic. You can supplement with garlic capsules but adding it to your food is the easiest method, and it'll make just about anything taste better.

1. Place potatoes in a slow cooker, adding enough water to cover them. Add salt and cook on low 4 hours or until potatoes are soft.

2. In a small saucepan over medium heat, sauté garlic in butter for 3 minutes or until garlic is slightly browned, and then stir in milk and sour cream, mixing well.

3. Drain potatoes and return to slow cooker, adding sauce. Mash with a potato masher or with a blender until smooth.

Per Serving | Calories: 131 | Fat: 3 g | Protein: 3 g | Sodium: 539 mg | Fiber: 3 g | Carbohydrates: 23 g | Sugar: 6 g

Cabbage Slaw

This low-calorie side is packed with healthy nutrients and fiber to keep you full and healthy.

INGREDIENTS | SERVES 4

½ small head cabbage, shredded

½ medium red bell pepper, seeded and sliced

¼ small red onion, peeled and sliced

2 tablespoons olive oil

5 teaspoons apple cider vinegar

¼ teaspoon salt

Moisten Your Cabbage with Salt

While shredded, fresh cabbage seems very dry and bland, it actually has a very high moisture content. Salt pulls water from things, so when you mix salt into your cabbage and let it sit for a while, you'll notice all sorts of juices coming out of the cabbage. Using salt is an easy, zero-calorie way to add some flavor and moisture to your cabbage dishes.

Toss all ingredients in a large bowl until mixed well and allow to chill at least 15 minutes in the refrigerator before serving.

Per Serving | Calories: 96 | Fat: 7 g | Protein: 2 g | Sodium: 167 mg | Fiber: 3 g | Carbohydrates: 8 g | Sugar: 5 g

Garlic Parmesan Fries

This recipe makes enough to serve two people, but you can prepare it in bulk to have on hand for the rest of the week or to feed a large party.

INGREDIENTS | SERVES 2

1 teaspoon olive oil
1 clove garlic, crushed
1 large potato, cut into fries
½ teaspoon salt
1 tablespoon grated Parmesan cheese
1 tablespoon chopped parsley

Bake Your Way to Better Health

French fries are traditionally, well, fried. The frying process can add trans fats and omega-6 fatty acids, which can cause inflammation and should be avoided. When you slice your fresh potatoes up and crisp them in the oven instead, you have a healthy side dish that's still delicious. Try mixing up your seasonings for variety—spicy seasonings, garlic salt, and ranch seasonings all work very well with homemade french fries.

1. Preheat oven to 425°F.

2. In a medium bowl, combine oil and garlic and toss potatoes in mixture, coating well.

3. Arrange fries on a baking sheet, spreading evenly, and top with salt. Bake 10 minutes per side.

4. Remove, top with Parmesan and parsley, and serve.

Per Serving | Calories: 163 | Fat: 3 g | Protein: 4 g | Sodium: 669 mg | Fiber: 5 g | Carbohydrates: 30 g | Sugar: 2 g

Cilantro Lime Low-Carb Rice

Using riced cauliflower is a great substitute for traditional rice recipes when you need to lower your daily carb intake.

INGREDIENTS | SERVES 4

1 (10-ounce) bag riced cauliflower (thawed or fresh)

3 tablespoons water

1 medium lime, juiced and zested

½ cup chopped cilantro

Low-Carb Rice at Home

Cauliflower is fairly neutral in flavor, particularly when you add other flavors and seasonings to it. If you're unable to find riced cauliflower at your local store, it's quite easy to make at home. Simply take a head of cauliflower, chop it up into bits, and run it through the food processor until well-chopped. You can steam up these little bits as a low-carb rice substitute.

1. Combine riced cauliflower and water in a large microwave-safe bowl and microwave 3–5 minutes or until cauliflower is soft.

2. Remove and add lime juice, zest, and cilantro to bowl. Mix well before serving.

Per Serving | Calories: 176 | Fat: 2 g | Protein: 14 g | Sodium: 170 mg | Fiber: 17 g | Carbohydrates: 35 g | Sugar: 16 g

Roasted Butternut Squash

*Butternut squash is similar to sweet potato in that it packs a lot of fiber,
as well as plenty of micronutrients for your health.*

INGREDIENTS | SERVES 4

1 medium butternut squash, peeled and cubed

2 tablespoons olive oil

2 cloves garlic, minced

1 teaspoon salt

1. Preheat oven to 400°F.

2. In a large bowl, toss squash, oil, and garlic until well coated. Spread on a baking sheet and season with salt.

3. Roast 25–30 minutes or until squash has browned.

Per Serving | Calories: 139 | Fat: 7 g | Protein: 2 g | Sodium: 589 mg | Fiber: 3 g | Carbohydrates: 20 g | Sugar: 4 g

Sweet Potato Fries

Sweet potato fries are the perfect way to enjoy this healthy starchy carb,
and this recipe bakes them to avoid the extra fat from traditional frying.

INGREDIENTS | SERVES 4

4 medium sweet potatoes, cut into fries
1 tablespoon water
2 teaspoons Italian seasoning
½ teaspoon lemon pepper
2 tablespoons olive oil
1 teaspoon salt
1 teaspoon freshly ground black pepper

1. Preheat oven to 400°F.

2. Combine all ingredients in a large bowl, tossing until potatoes are well coated. Arrange on a baking sheet.

3. Cook 30 minutes, turning halfway through, until fries reach desired level of crispness.

Per Serving | Calories: 160 | Fat: 7 g | Protein: 2 g | Sodium: 645 mg | Fiber: 4 g | Carbohydrates: 24 g | Sugar: 5 g

Garlic and Lemon Jasmine Rice

Jasmine rice may be the tastiest rice available, and it's sticky and easy to eat. This unique lemon and garlic twist on jasmine rice makes a refreshing side dish.

INGREDIENTS | SERVES 2

1 cup uncooked jasmine rice

1 tablespoon olive oil

3 cloves garlic, minced

½ teaspoon salt

2 teaspoons chopped parsley

1 teaspoon lemon juice

1. Prepare rice on stove or in rice cooker according to package directions.

2. Add oil, garlic, salt, parsley, and lemon to cooked rice, mix well, and serve warm.

Per Serving | Calories: 405 | Fat: 7 g | Protein: 7 g | Sodium: 588 mg | Fiber: 1 g | Carbohydrates: 76 g | Sugar: 0 g

Buffalo and Blue Cheese Brussels Sprouts

If you want a meat-free and low-fat version of buffalo wings for the big game, these brussels sprouts are a healthy alternative to fried wings.

INGREDIENTS | SERVES 4

2 tablespoons olive oil

1 pound brussels sprouts, trimmed and halved

¼ cup Franks RedHot Original Cayenne Pepper Sauce

2 tablespoons blue cheese crumbles

Fire Up Your Metabolism with Hot Sauce

Hot sauce contains capsaicin, which may slightly increase your metabolism. Adding hot sauce to your meals won't be enough to make you lose a lot of weight, but it certainly can't hurt anything, and it makes your food taste better. If you're low on calories and want to keep your metabolism up, eating spicy foods may be just what you need.

1. Preheat oven to 425°F.

2. While oven heats, sauté brussels sprouts in oil in a large skillet over medium heat about 5 minutes until softened.

3. Spread on a baking sheet and roast in the oven an additional 10–12 minutes.

4. Transfer to a large bowl, toss with hot sauce until well coated, and top with blue cheese crumbles before serving.

Per Serving | Calories: 123 | Fat: 8 g | Protein: 5 g | Sodium: 639 mg | Fiber: 4 g | Carbohydrates: 10 g | Sugar: 3 g

Zucchini Fries

If you want a crispy fry recipe without the carbs from potatoes, zucchinis make an excellent substitution.

INGREDIENTS | SERVES 4

1 cup bread crumbs

¼ teaspoon garlic powder

2 tablespoons grated Parmesan cheese

¼ teaspoon salt

3 large egg whites, beaten

4 medium zucchinis, peeled and cut into fries

1. Preheat oven to 425°F.

2. Combine bread crumbs, garlic, cheese, and salt in a large bowl. Place egg whites in a separate bowl.

3. Dip zucchini sticks into egg whites, toss in bread crumb mixture to coat, and arrange on a greased baking sheet.

4. Bake 20 minutes or until fries begin to brown, turning halfway through.

Per Serving | Calories: 165 | Fat: 3 g | Protein: 10 g | Sodium: 445 mg | Fiber: 3 g | Carbohydrates: 27 g | Sugar: 6 g

CHAPTER 13

Snacks

Cinnamon Apple Protein Bars

If you rely on protein bars as healthy snacks, you'll love this healthy, homemade recipe. Say goodbye to stomach cramps from weird protein bar ingredients and say hello to your new healthy recipe.

INGREDIENTS | SERVES 4

¾ cup dry oats

¼ cup oat bran

6 large egg whites

1 scoop vanilla protein powder

2 tablespoons unsweetened applesauce

¼ teaspoon baking powder

1 packet stevia

1 teaspoon cinnamon

2 tablespoons olive oil

2 medium apples, diced

1. Preheat oven to 350°F.

2. Combine all ingredients except apples in blender until well mixed.

3. Pour into a large bowl, add apples, and mix well.

4. Spread mixture in a 10" × 13" lightly greased glass baking dish and bake 30 minutes.

5. Cut into 4 equal squares and allow to cool.

Per Serving | Calories: 170 | Fat: 2 g | Protein: 15 g | Sodium: 43 mg | Fiber: 4 g | Carbohydrates: 27 g | Sugar: 10 g

Save Your Gut with Homemade Bars

To save calories, many popular protein bars on the market use various sugar alcohols and other additives to add flavor without using actual sugar. It's very common for these ingredients to cause digestive pain and cramping. If you've ever eaten a protein bar and noticed discomfort, there's a good chance it was the sugar alcohols, not the protein itself.

Cinnamon Protein Apple Slices

This two-minute recipe is reminiscent of apple pie but provides the healthy, filling combination of apples and protein.

INGREDIENTS | SERVES 1

½ scoop vanilla protein powder

1 packet stevia or other sweetener

2 teaspoons cinnamon

1 medium apple, sliced

1. Combine protein, stevia, and cinnamon in a sandwich bag or bowl.

2. Add apple slices, tossing until coated, and serve.

Per Serving | Calories: 90 | Fat: 0 g | Protein: 1 g | Sodium: 1 mg | Fiber: 5 g | Carbohydrates: 25 g | Sugar: 16 g

Protein Sludge

The easiest way to consume protein powder without having to choke down a protein shake—sludge may be the most versatile protein recipe out there.

INGREDIENTS | SERVES 1

1½ scoops whey protein, any flavor
¼ cup frozen mixed berries
2 tablespoons water

1. Place protein powder in a small bowl.

2. Add a splash of water, stir well, and repeat until protein is the consistency of a thick pudding.

3. Top with mixed berries.

Per Serving | Calories: 190 | Fat: 1 g | Protein: 40 g | Sodium: 65 mg | Fiber: 1 g | Carbohydrates: 7 g | Sugar: 5 g

Sludge for the Macros

Protein sludge sounds really bad. It's not. By mixing protein and water, you can make a delicious, pudding-style protein treat and avoid choking down another chalky shake. Best of all, you can customize the recipe any way you want. Use different flavors of protein to see what you like, and if you need some fat or carbs, try adding oats, nut butters, berries, whipped cream, or anything else you can dream of.

Café Mocha Protein Bars

This version of a protein bar combines the flavors of chocolate and coffee for a rich, invigorating, and protein-packed snack.

INGREDIENTS | SERVES 4

¾ cup dry oatmeal

¼ cup oat bran

6 large egg whites

1 scoop chocolate protein powder

¼ teaspoon baking powder

1 teaspoon cocoa powder

1 tablespoon ground coffee

1 packet stevia

1. Preheat oven to 350°F.

2. Combine all ingredients in a blender and mix until smooth, then transfer to a greased 10" × 13" baking dish.

3. Bake 30 minutes and allow to cool before serving, cutting into 4 equal bars.

Per Serving | Calories: 127 | Fat: 2 g | Protein: 15 g | Sodium: 42 mg | Fiber: 3 g | Carbohydrates: 15 g | Sugar: 1 g

Is It Okay to Bake with Protein?

You may have read that baking protein "denatures" it, rendering it useless. Exposing whey protein to high heat can indeed denature it, but this doesn't make it worthless; it just changes its molecular structure. In other words, your food might taste a little dry if you use too much powder, but you're still getting all the benefits of the protein.

Easy Kale Chips

Kale is the healthiest green on the planet, but it can be quite bitter to eat raw. Making kale chips is super easy and results in an addicting and healthy snack.

INGREDIENTS | SERVES 2

2 cups raw kale leaves, washed and torn into smaller pieces

1 tablespoon olive oil

2 teaspoons garlic salt

1 tablespoon grated Parmesan cheese

1. Preheat oven to 400°F.

2. Dry kale thoroughly using paper towels or a salad spinner; mix it with oil in a large bowl, coating each piece well.

3. Spread kale out evenly over baking sheet covered with aluminum foil.

4. Sprinkle with garlic salt and Parmesan.

5. Bake 8–12 minutes or until it reaches your desired crispness.

Per Serving | Calories: 81 | Fat: 8 g | Protein: 2 g | Sodium: 2,023 mg | Fiber: 1 g | Carbohydrates: 2 g | Sugar: 0 g

Chai Latte Power Shake

If you love chai, you'll love this filling protein smoothie. The added caffeine from the chai tea also serves as a nice afternoon pick-me-up to get you through the day.

INGREDIENTS | SERVES 1

1 scoop vanilla protein powder
1 cup cold cinnamon chai tea
1 packet stevia
1 teaspoon cinnamon
5 ice cubes

Place all ingredients in a blender and blend until smooth. Serve immediately.

Per Serving | Calories: 119 | Fat: 0 g | Protein: 27 g | Sodium: 43 mg | Fiber: 1 g | Carbohydrates: 3 g | Sugar: 1 g

The Best Protein Powder for Recipes

Protein powder is very useful for hitting your protein macronutrient quota, but it's not all created equal. It's important to get your protein from a reputable brand as several companies have been caught lying about what's on their labels. Do your research and find a company you trust. For recipes, whey protein is the most versatile, and having vanilla and/or chocolate gives you a safe, neutral flavor that goes well with just about anything.

Shamrock Shake Protein Smoothie

This cold, minty, refreshing protein smoothie tastes like a milkshake—a healthy one.

INGREDIENTS | SERVES 1

1 scoop chocolate protein powder

1 teaspoon mint extract

½ cup skim milk

1 cup cold water

1 teaspoon cocoa powder

1 packet stevia

5 ice cubes

Place all ingredients in a blender and blend until smooth. Serve immediately.

Per Serving | Calories: 180 | Fat: 2 g | Protein: 31 g | Sodium: 104 mg | Fiber: 1 g | Carbohydrates: 9 g | Sugar: 8 g

Kefir and Chia Super Pudding

Kefir is loaded with probiotics and good bacteria.
When combined with chia seeds, a superfood, it makes for a very healthy snack.

INGREDIENTS | SERVES 2

1 cup plain kefir
1 cup mixed berries
3 tablespoons chia seeds
½ cup unsweetened almond milk

What Is Kefir, Anyway?

Many believe that kefir is similar to quality yogurts because it contains healthy probiotics that are good for your gut. This is true, but there's more to the story. Kefir also contains yeast and the types of good bacteria that can actually remain in your gut and help you maintain a healthy digestive environment. In contrast, regular yogurt just passes through without providing many benefits.

1. Place kefir and berries in a blender and blend until smooth.

2. Pour mixture into a large bowl and stir in chia seeds and almond milk. Allow to set in the refrigerator at least 6 hours before serving.

Per Serving | Calories: 205 | Fat: 8 g | Protein: 10 g | Sodium: 109 mg | Fiber: 9 g | Carbohydrates: 26 g | Sugar: 13 g

Homemade Tortilla Chips

*Everyone loves chips and salsa, and this quick and easy homemade recipe
gives you peace of mind about what you're eating.*

INGREDIENTS | SERVES 6

10 medium corn tortillas
3 tablespoons lime juice
1 tablespoon olive oil
1 teaspoon salt

1. Preheat oven to 350°F.

2. Cut tortillas into chip-sized pieces and spread evenly on a lightly oiled baking sheet.

3. Mix lime juice and oil in a small bowl and brush or spray on tortillas, then lightly salt tortillas.

4. Cook 12–14 minutes or until crispy, turning halfway through.

Per Serving | Calories: 109 | Fat: 3 g | Protein: 2 g | Sodium: 407 mg | Fiber: 3 g | Carbohydrates: 18 g | Sugar: 1 g

Classic Deviled Eggs

Deviled eggs are a popular snack, very healthy, and quite easy to make.
Bring these to a party or make in bulk and store for later use.

INGREDIENTS | SERVES 8

4 large hard-boiled eggs, peeled and cut in half lengthwise

1 tablespoon mustard

1 tablespoon mayonnaise

½ teaspoon garlic salt

½ teaspoon onion powder

1 teaspoon paprika

1. Scoop yolks out of egg white halves into a medium bowl.

2. Combine mustard, mayonnaise, garlic salt, and onion powder with yolks and mix well.

3. Scoop mixture into hollowed-out egg white halves, top with paprika, and refrigerate until ready to serve.

Per Serving | Calories: 51 | Fat: 4 g | Protein: 3 g | Sodium: 189 mg | Fiber: 0 g | Carbohydrates: 1 g | Sugar: 0 g

How to Make Easy-to-Peel Hard-Boiled Eggs

The most annoying part of eating hard-boiled eggs is the peeling process. It can be tough to peel the eggs without removing half the egg white along with the shell. To make this easier, add about a tablespoon of vinegar to your boiling water. Also, cool the eggs as quickly as possible after cooking by moving them to a bowl filled with ice water instead of just running them under tap water.

Homemade Hummus

Hummus is a delicious snack, an excellent source of healthy fats, and very easy to make at home with the right ingredients.

INGREDIENTS | SERVES 12

1 (15-ounce) can chickpeas, drained (reserve liquid in a bowl)

2 tablespoons tahini paste

2 tablespoons lemon juice

2 cloves garlic, minced

¾ teaspoon salt

1. Combine all ingredients in a blender, including 2 tablespoons of reserved bean liquid, and blend until smooth.

2. Transfer to a medium bowl and store covered in the refrigerator until ready to eat.

Per Serving | Calories: 45 | Fat: 2 g | Protein: 2 g | Sodium: 252 mg | Fiber: 2 g | Carbohydrates: 7 g | Sugar: 0 g

Classic Granola

Granola packs a lot of calories in a small serving, so if you have a busy schedule that doesn't allow you to sit down for big meals, granola is a filling and energizing snack.

INGREDIENTS | SERVES 12

3 cups dry oats

1 cup coconut flakes

1 cup almonds or mixed nuts

5 tablespoons coconut oil, melted

1 teaspoon vanilla extract

¼ teaspoon salt

1 cup dried berries

Granola: Healthy but High in Calories

Granola is one of the healthiest snacks you can eat, but it's high in fat and very easy to overeat. It's definitely healthy fat, but this fat makes granola very dense in calories. If you're trying to lose weight, measure out your granola and leave the rest at home so you don't accidentally eat half the bag—something that's very easy to do with such a delicious snack.

1. Preheat oven to 350°F.

2. Combine oats, coconut, almonds, oil, vanilla, and salt in a large bowl, mixing well before spreading on a baking sheet lined with parchment paper.

3. Bake 20–25 minutes or until granola is golden brown, turning halfway through.

4. Remove and allow to cool. Mix with dried fruit and store in an airtight container.

Per Serving | Calories: 238 | Fat: 16 g | Protein: 6 g | Sodium: 52 mg | Fiber: 5 g | Carbohydrates: 19 g | Sugar: 2 g

CHAPTER 14

Desserts

Protein Fluff

This delicious treat is very filling and will keep you feeling satisfied and energized.
Use any combinations of protein and berries that you prefer.
Whey protein will work in this recipe but won't "fluff" as well as the casein.

INGREDIENTS | SERVES 2

½ cup frozen berries, slightly thawed

2 scoops chocolate casein protein

¼ cup skim milk

1 packet stevia or your sweetener of choice

What Is Protein Fluff?

By mixing all the ingredients in a bowl, you already have a satisfying, filling treat. If you have a blender available, however, mixing it for 5–10 minutes can double or even triple the volume, making this taste like fruity whipped cream. You may actually find it hard to avoid eating the entire bowl, so it's a great way to fill your stomach with very few calories.

1. Add all ingredients in a medium bowl and stir. The mixture should have a thick, pudding-like texture. (You can eat it now as is or continue to next step to make it fluffy.)

2. Using a power blender, blend mixture on medium 5–10 minutes until it fluffs up.

Per Serving | Calories: 116 | Fat: 1 g | Protein: 20 g | Sodium: 64 mg | Fiber: 1 g | Carbohydrates: 8 g | Sugar: 5 g

Triple Berry Yogurt Parfait

This is a fun and sweet treat that's perfect for a relaxing day.
You can choose high- or low-fat ingredients to make this fit your caloric goals.

INGREDIENTS | SERVES 2

1 cup vanilla Greek yogurt

½ cup fresh blueberries

½ cup fresh blackberries

½ cup fresh raspberries

½ cup fat-free whipped cream

½ cup granola or high-fiber cereal

In a glass or small bowl, layer the ingredients in a visually pleasing manner or mix it all up to enjoy.

Per Serving | Calories: 238 | Fat: 5 g | Protein: 15 g | Sodium: 56 mg | Fiber: 7 g | Carbohydrates: 38 g | Sugar: 23 g

Berries: Micronutrient Bombs

Berries are very rich in vitamins, minerals, and antioxidants that help your body flush out all the bad free radicals produced by stress. They are also high in fiber and support healthy digestion. In addition, their natural sugars help satisfy your sweet tooth.

Frozen Chocolate Banana

The perfect summer treat, quick to prepare and easy to grab and enjoy.

INGREDIENTS | SERVES 2

2 medium bananas

4 onces dark chocolate

½ cup ground peanuts, or any topping you prefer

Bananas for Exercise

When you are very active, especially during the summer months, it's very important to stay hydrated, as you can sweat out electrolytes. Bananas are not only a great source of natural sugar, they are full of potassium to keep you hydrated and help prevent cramping.

1. Peel bananas, cut in half, and place in freezer until firm.

2. Melt dark chocolate in a bowl in the microwave 3–5 minutes or until soft, or over the stove until soft.

3. Remove bananas from freezer and roll them in melted chocolate to cover, sprinkle with nuts or topping of choice, and return to the freezer until ready to enjoy.

Per Serving | Calories: 580 | Fat: 35 g | Protein: 13 g | Sodium: 13 mg | Fiber: 9 g | Carbohydrates: 68 g | Sugar: 46 g

Peanut Butter Protein Cookies

The protein and fat in this recipe will keep you full with minimal carbohydrates.
It's perfect for your sweet tooth on those low-carb days.

INGREDIENTS | MAKES 10 COOKIES

1 cup natural peanut butter
2 large egg whites
1 scoop vanilla protein powder
¾ cup stevia
1 teaspoon cinnamon

Cycle Your Nut Sources

Nuts are one of the best natural sources of fat available and even contain a little bit of protein. If you get tired of regular peanut butter, try cycling your nut butters. Almond butter, cashew butter, and even sunflower seed butter are all delicious and healthy options you can use for variety.

1. Preheat oven to 350°F.

2. Place all ingredients into a medium bowl and stir.

3. Shape dough into round cookies and spread out on a greased cookie sheet, leaving 1" between cookies.

4. Bake 10 minutes, cool, and serve.

Per Serving (1 cookie) | Calories: 168 | Fat: 13 g | Protein: 8 g | Sodium: 95 mg | Fiber: 2 g | Carbohydrates: 8 g | Sugar: 3 g

High-Protein Oatmeal Cookies

This cookie recipe brings the carbs and protein with very little fat.
The oatmeal also provides fiber, which will help keep you feeling full.
These cookies are great for when you need a low-fat, sustained energy boost.

INGREDIENTS | MAKES 12 COOKIES

1¾ cups dry oats
4 scoops vanilla protein powder
½ cup applesauce
½ cup egg whites
1 tablespoon olive oil
1 tablespoon stevia
Dash cinnamon

1. Preheat oven to 350°F.

2. Place ingredients in a large bowl and stir.

3. Shape dough into round cookies and spread out on a greased cookie sheet 1" apart.

4. Bake 10–15 minutes, until lightly browned.

Per Serving (1 cookie) | Calories: 149 | Fat: 4 g | Protein: 9 g | Sodium: 46 mg | Fiber: 5 g | Carbohydrates: 21 g | Sugar: 2 g

Protein Cheesecake

Cheesecake is notorious for being a high-fat recipe, but this version is incredibly low in fat with a high protein content and delicious flavor. Top with berries for an extra sweet nutritional treat.

INGREDIENTS | MAKES 1 CHEESECAKE (SERVES 12)

24 ounces fat-free cream cheese

2 scoops vanilla whey protein

¾ cup stevia

1 teaspoon vanilla extract

3 large eggs

1 tablespoon lemon juice

Use Flavored Proteins in Your Baking

Most recipes can be made with chocolate or vanilla protein powders, which are readily available just about anywhere and are generally mild-flavored and safe to use. If you're feeling a little adventurous, head to your local supplement shop and check out their selection. You can often find many more flavors than you'd find at your grocery store if you want to move beyond chocolate and vanilla.

1. Preheat oven to 350°F.

2. Place ingredients in a large bowl and mix with a hand mixer on medium speed.

3. Pour mix into a 9" pie pan coated with nonstick cooking spray.

4. Bake 45 minutes and refrigerate 3 hours or until ready to serve.

Per Serving | Calories: 177 | Fat: 3 g | Protein: 24 g | Sodium: 800 mg | Fiber: 0 g | Carbohydrates: 11 g | Sugar: 7 g

Peanut Butter Banana Frozen Greek Yogurt

This super quick, super delicious treat is perfect for satisfying your sweet tooth with natural ingredients. If you want to experiment with flavors, take out the protein and add lemon juice for a tart treat, or frozen berries.

INGREDIENTS | SERVES 1

½ cup Greek yogurt

1 medium frozen banana, sliced

2 tablespoons natural peanut butter

Blend all ingredients in a blender or food processor until smooth and serve immediately.

Per Serving | Calories: 362 | Fat: 16 g | Protein: 20 g | Sodium: 139 mg | Fiber: 5 g | Carbohydrates: 41 g | Sugar: 23 g

No-Bake Cookie Bites

This is a quick and healthy alternative to chocolate chip cookies, using only five ingredients to make these delicious snacks.

INGREDIENTS | MAKES 8 COOKIES

1 cup dry oats
1 cup raw almonds
10 Medjool dates, pitted
½ cup water
¼ cup chocolate chips

1. Blend oats and almonds in a food processor until powdered.

2. Add dates and continue to blend until mixed well.

3. Continue to blend while slowly adding water until a thick paste texture forms.

4. Stir in chocolate chips, roll into bite-sized portions, place on lined baking sheet, and refrigerate until ready to serve.

Per Serving (1 cookie) | Calories: 266 | Fat: 12 g | Protein: 6 g | Sodium: 0 mg | Fiber: 6 g | Carbohydrates: 36 g | Sugar: 25 g

Three Ingredient Cinnamon Pecan Bites

Minimal ingredients provide a great source of healthy fats for sustained energy, and the end result is delicious and easy to prepare.

INGREDIENTS | MAKES 10–12 COOKIES

10 pitted dates, soaked in water 15 minutes

2 cups raw pecans

2 teaspoons cinnamon

Bake with Dates

Dates may not be a popular snack, but these sticky-sweet treats make a great natural sweetener for your baking needs. In addition to adding natural sugars, dates can add moisture and fiber, giving your recipes extra richness and flavor without the need for sugar and butter.

1. Preheat oven to 350°F.

2. Drain dates and combine all ingredients in food processor, blending until smooth.

3. Shape into small balls and place on lined cooking sheets 1" apart.

4. Bake 10–12 minutes and allow to cool before serving.

Per Serving (1 cookie) | Calories: 228 | Fat: 16 g | Protein: 3 g | Sodium: 0 mg | Fiber: 4 g | Carbohydrates: 22 g | Sugar: 17 g

Vanilla Peach Protein Bars

*These bars provide protein, carbs, fiber, and very little fat,
making a sweet, tasty, and refreshing dessert.*

INGREDIENTS | SERVES 4

¾ cup dry oats

¼ cup oat bran

6 large egg whites

1 scoop vanilla protein powder

¼ teaspoon baking powder

¼ teaspoon stevia

2 tablespoons olive oil

Drop vanilla extract

2 medium peaches, peeled and diced

1. Preheat oven to 350°F.

2. In a blender, mix all ingredients except peaches and transfer to a large bowl.

3. Add peaches to mixture, stirring to combine.

4. Pour the mixture into a lightly greased 10" × 13" baking dish and bake 30 minutes. Cut into 4 bars when cooled.

Per Serving | Calories: 147 | Fat: 1 g | Protein: 18 g | Sodium: 114 mg | Fiber: 2 g | Carbohydrates: 19 g | Sugar: 5 g

Summer Fruit Salad

Fruit is the perfect natural sweetner, containing natural sugars that your body will love. Adding some yogurt provides just a touch of sweetness and protein.

INGREDIENTS | SERVES 4

2 cups strawberries, sliced

1 pound seedless grapes, halved

3 medium bananas, peeled and sliced

1 (12-ounce) container low-fat strawberry yogurt or flavor of your choice

Mix all ingredients together in a large bowl and chill until ready to serve.

Per Serving | Calories: 211 | Fat: 1 g | Protein: 5 g | Sodium: 18 mg | Fiber: 5 g | Carbohydrates: 52 g | Sugar: 38 g

Apple Crisp Bowls

Apple crisp is delicious but takes time to make and is usually very high in calories. This alternative and healthy recipe provides a delicious, lower-calorie option for when you're craving a delicious apple treat.

INGREDIENTS | SERVES 1

¾ cup Greek yogurt

2 tablespoons unsweetened applesauce

1 medium apple, peeled and diced

¼ teaspoon stevia

¼ teaspoon cinnamon

¼ teaspoon nutmeg

Mix all ingredients together in a small bowl and serve.

Per Serving | Calories: 187 | Fat: 0 g | Protein: 19 g | Sodium: 90 mg | Fiber: 6 g | Carbohydrates: 33 g | Sugar: 25 g

An Apple a Day Keeps the Hunger Away

Apples are one of the best fruits to enjoy on a diet. Not only do they come in a variety of shapes, sizes, and flavors, but they are also an excellent natural source of pectin. Pectin, like fiber, helps you feel full and satisfied. So if you're feeling hungry between meals, an apple is the perfect snack to hold you over until the next meal.

Protein-Packed Banana Pudding

This pudding recipe uses high-protein ingredients with the sweetness of a banana to bring it all together. If you want a tasty, creamy dessert you can enjoy guilt-free, make this in bulk and keep on hand for when that sweet tooth strikes.

INGREDIENTS | SERVES 2

¾ cup low-fat Greek yogurt
1 teaspoon fat-free sour cream
½ scoop vanilla protein powder
1 medium banana, sliced
½ packet stevia

Mix all ingredients together in a small bowl and chill until ready to eat.

Per Serving | Calories: 142 | Fat: 0 g | Protein: 14 g | Sodium: 54 mg | Fiber: 2 g | Carbohydrates: 20 g | Sugar: 12 g

Neapolitan Smoothie

Everyone loves Neapolitan milkshakes, but nobody wants the insanely high calories that come along with it. This simple smoothie combines chocolate, vanilla, and strawberry, along with a high protein count, making it an ideal dessert or post-workout shake.

INGREDIENTS | SERVES 1

1 scoop vanilla protein powder

4 frozen strawberries

1 teaspoon cocoa powder

1 teaspoon sugar-free Hershey's chocolate syrup

1 packet stevia

3–4 ice cubes

In a blender, blend all ingredients until smooth. Serve immediately.

Per Serving | Calories: 141 | Fat: 1 g | Protein: 21 g | Sodium: 66 mg | Fiber: 2 g | Carbohydrates: 15 g | Sugar: 4 g

Strawberries and Cream

*This simple yet elegant dessert is quite easy to make and
is the perfect treat for a hot summer night.*

INGREDIENTS | SERVES 5

½ cup low-fat sour cream

2 tablespoons brown sugar or brown sugar substitute

1 pound fresh strawberries, cleaned and hulled

Stevia Substitutes

Stevia is the best natural sweetener as it's made from plants, not chemicals, and it's very sweet. If you check the baking aisle, you'll find all kinds of stevia, ranging from plain stevia packets, to brown sugar stevia substitutes, and even liquid stevia drops. If you want to cut the sugar without using chemical additives, stevia is the way to go.

1. Prepare the cream by combining sour cream and sugar substitute in a bowl, mixing well.

2. Place 5–6 strawberries in each dish and drizzle with about 2 tablespoons of the cream mixture before serving.

Per Serving | Calories: 75 | Fat: 2 g | Protein: 2 g | Sodium: 21 mg | Fiber: 2 g | Carbohydrates: 13 g | Sugar: 11 g

Creamy Coconut Popsicles

Coconuts are both a potent source of healthy fats and extremely hydrating. These treats are quick to prepare, and once frozen, they make a tasty and refreshing summer treat. If you want to lower the carbs, replace the powdered sugar with stevia instead.

INGREDIENTS | SERVES 10

1 (8-ounce) can evaporated skim milk

1 (8-ounce) can coconut milk

½ cup confectoners' sugar

½ teaspoon cinnamon

½ cup shredded coconut

1. Combine all ingredients in a large bowl and mix thoroughly.

2. Pour into your favorite popsicle molds, allow to freeze completely, and serve.

Per Serving | Calories: 102 | Fat: 4 g | Protein: 3 g | Sodium: 88 mg | Fiber: 1 g | Carbohydrates: 14 g | Sugar: 13 g

Tropical Fruit for Your Health

Tropical fruits like coconut, pineapple, papaya, and mango are very powerful health foods. They are tasty, sweet, and help aid in the digestion process, making you more efficient at breaking down and absorbing the food you eat.

Low-Fat Brownies

By replacing any oil, whole eggs, or butter with a can of black beans, this recipe provides a high-fiber, low-fat treat. It's not exactly low on calories, but it's perfect for high-carb days when fat needs to stay low.

INGREDIENTS | MAKES 20 BROWNIES

1 (15-ounce) can black beans, drained and rinsed

1 (19-ounce) box of your favorite brownie mix

1. Blend beans in a food processor until smooth.

2. Combine with package of brownie mix, transfer to an oiled 10" × 13" baking dish, and bake according to package directions.

Per Serving (1 brownie) | Calories: 121 | Fat: 1 g | Protein: 1 g | Sodium: 148 mg | Fiber: 1 g | Carbohydrates: 26 g | Sugar: 15 g

Tart Cheesecake Bites

This tart and healthy treat uses the refreshing taste of lemons to mimic the tartness of a traditional cheesecake, with a lot less fat and calories accompanying it.

INGREDIENTS | MAKES 12 BITES

12 reduced-fat vanilla wafers
8 ounces low-fat cream cheese, softened
¼ cup baking stevia
1 teaspoon vanilla extract
¾ cup low-fat Greek yogurt
3 tablespoons lemon juice
1 tablespoon lemon zest
2 large egg whites

1. Heat oven to 350°F.

2. Line a muffin tin with baking liners and place a single vanilla wafer into the bottom of each one.

3. Combine cream cheese, stevia, and vanilla in a medium bowl, using a mixer to blend until smooth.

4. Add yogurt, lemon juice, lemon zest, and egg whites and continue to blend until mixed well.

5. Pour evenly into baking liners, filling about halfway.

6. Bake 20–25 minutes and allow to cool in the refrigerator before serving.

Per Serving (1 bite) | Calories: 85 | Fat: 3 g | Protein: 4 g | Sodium: 101 mg | Fiber: 1 g | Carbohydrates: 7 g | Sugar: 4 g

CHAPTER 15

Two-Week Sample Meal Plan

The key to success is planning ahead and making things as easy as possible. If you simplify the process, you have the best chance of setting yourself up for success. Chapter 5 taught you how to build your own meal plan, but if you need some help or ideas, this chapter will provide some guidance. You'll notice that breakfast, lunch, and snacks often repeat themselves—this allows you to prepare food in advance and have it ready to go for later, saving you time during your busy week. Dinners rotate for variety. All of the recipes are in this book and all portions can be adjusted to fit your individual needs.

Week One

The sample weeks shown here follow a simple three-meal-per-day plan. You can use snacks or extra meals to target any macronutrients you may be missing. If you use this plan, be sure to adjust the portions to fit your daily macronutrient requirements. If you build your own, you can copy this format. Remember, the easier you make the plan, the easier it will be for you to stick to it. Eating the same meals throughout the week may seem boring, but it's one less thing you need to think about.

ESSENTIAL

While meal planning is a great tool, it isn't always realistic on a busy schedule. If you find that you eat different foods every single day, use a smartphone app to track your food intake. This way, you can always see in a matter of seconds how many calories you've consumed and how many you have remaining for the day.

Plan your week, make a list of what you need, and prep your food on Sunday. This is the easiest way to make sure you have no excuses to stray from your plan during the week.

Having things planned ahead also makes it easier to plan indulgences. If you have a social event or a lunch outing, simply replace that meal in your plan, look at how it affects your daily macros, and plan around that meal accordingly.

SUNDAY

- **Breakfast:** Island Breakfast Bowl (Chapter 6)
- **Lunch:** Buffalo Chicken Mini Wraps (Chapter 7)
- **Dinner:** Seared Chilean Sea Bass with Homemade Pesto (Chapter 9)

MONDAY

- **Breakfast:** Breakfast Bake (Chapter 6)
- **Lunch:** Tuna Salad (Chapter 7)
- **Dinner:** Pesto Chili (Chapter 8)

TUESDAY

- **Breakfast:** Island Breakfast Bowl (Chapter 6)
- **Lunch:** Buffalo Chicken Mini Wraps (Chapter 7)
- **Dinner:** Pasta with Pesto and Olive Sauce (Chapter 8)

WEDNESDAY

- **Breakfast:** Breakfast Bake (Chapter 6)
- **Lunch:** Tuna Salad (Chapter 7)
- **Dinner:** Clam Chowder (Chapter 9)

THURSDAY

- **Breakfast:** Island Breakfast Bowl (Chapter 6)
- **Lunch:** Buffalo Chicken Mini Wraps (Chapter 7)
- **Dinner:** Southwestern Fajitas (Chapter 10)

FRIDAY

- **Breakfast:** Breakfast Bake (Chapter 6)
- **Lunch:** Tuna Salad (Chapter 7)
- **Dinner:** Seared Tilapia with Pan Sauce (Chapter 9)

SATURDAY

- **Breakfast:** Island Breakfast Bowl (Chapter 6)
- **Lunch:** Buffalo Chicken Mini Wraps (Chapter 7)
- **Dinner:** Black Bean Soup (Chapter 8)

Week Two

SUNDAY

- **Breakfast:** Maple Pecan Banana Muffins (Chapter 6)
- **Lunch:** Turkey Reuben Sandwiches (Chapter 7)
- **Dinner:** Lemon-Herb Grilled Chicken Salad (Chapter 10)

MONDAY

- **Breakfast:** Banana Pancakes (Chapter 6)
- **Lunch:** Chipotle Lime Cod Fillets (Chapter 7)
- **Dinner:** Shrimp Taco Salad (Chapter 9)

TUESDAY

- **Breakfast:** Maple Pecan Banana Muffins (Chapter 6)
- **Lunch:** Turkey Reuben Sandwiches (Chapter 7)
- **Dinner:** Pulled-Chicken BBQ Sandwiches (Chapter 10)

WEDNESDAY

- **Breakfast:** Banana Pancakes (Chapter 6)
- **Lunch:** Chipotle Lime Cod Fillets (Chapter 7)
- **Dinner:** Maryland Crab Cakes (Chapter 9)

THURSDAY

- **Breakfast:** Maple Pecan Banana Muffins (Chapter 6)
- **Lunch:** Turkey Reuben Sandwiches (Chapter 7)
- **Dinner:** Greek Butterflied Chicken (Chapter 10)

FRIDAY

- **Breakfast:** Banana Pancakes (Chapter 6)
- **Lunch:** Chipotle Lime Cod Fillets (Chapter 7)
- **Dinner:** Chicken and Bean Protein Burritos (Chapter 10)

SATURDAY

- **Breakfast:** Maple Pecan Banana Muffins (Chapter 6)
- **Lunch:** Turkey Reuben Sandwiches (Chapter 7)
- **Dinner:** Tuscan-Style Slow Cooker Chicken (Chapter 10)

APPENDIX A

Frequently Asked Questions

How does alcohol affect my diet?

From a purely caloric perspective, it's possible to fit alcohol into your diet. Since alcohol provides no nutritional value, you simply take the total calories in your drinks and subtract them from your carbohydrate and fat calories. You can drink, but you'll just have to eat less.

The biggest concern for fat loss is typically eating while intoxicated. After a couple of drinks, you may have a harder time saying no to foods you wouldn't otherwise eat. Also, since alcohol is a toxin, your metabolism can shift to burning alcohol for energy to remove it from your body, meaning most of the food you eat and digest would get stored as fat rather than used as energy. To be safe, try to drink plenty of water when consuming alcohol and eat a healthy snack beforehand so you don't end up hungry and intoxicated.

Are supplements necessary?

You don't need any supplements at all to lose weight. Certain supplements, like protein, fish oil, and vitamin D, can be very useful for overall health, but you can get enough from your diet if it's properly structured. If you're curious about a supplement, use Examine.com to find unbiased research reviews from doctors who will tell you if a given ingredient works, and if so, how much to use.

For an up-to-date list of supplements the author uses and recommends in his fitness coaching business, visit www.mattdustin.com/macronutrients.

How fast can I lose weight?

Ideally, you shouldn't lose more than 1 percent of your body weight each week. For most people this works out to 1–2 pounds of fat loss per week, but it could be more or less depending on how much you weigh.

Your body is smart and will always seek balance. It doesn't like to lose weight too quickly, so if you drop your calories extremely low overnight to lose weight, your body will fight to slow down weight loss and adjust. Typically when someone loses a lot of weight very quickly and then goes off their diet, it's very common for that person to put all of the weight back on and then some.

Fat loss should be a slow, steady process so that you can build good habits along the way that you'll be able to sustain for life. The goal should always be to do as little as possible; that is, eat as much as possible while still making progress. Every time progress stalls, you'll have to lower your food intake or add more exercise, so you want to leave yourself as much room to work with as possible.

If you immediately adopt a very low caloric intake, you won't be able to adjust much when progress stalls without making yourself miserable. Take it slow and steady and let your body do its thing.

The one time that rapid weight loss is okay is when you initially start a diet. It's very common to lose anywhere from 5–10 pounds in the first week, but it's usually just excess water weight you're dropping from cleaning up your diet. Once your body adjusts to the new plan, 1–2 pounds per week is a more appropriate and manageable goal.

What happens if I just can't lose weight, no matter how low my calories go?

In rare cases, you might actually be stuck. If your calories are extremely low—usually 1,000–1,200 is about the lowest you want to safely go—and you're exercising on a regular basis, you should be losing fat. Double-check everything with your diet. You may find hidden calories in what you drink, snacks you eat, or condiments you use. Oftentimes stubborn fat comes off eventually; it just takes a lot of work and self-discipline.

If you're 100 percent sure your diet is accurate, you're active, and your body just isn't losing weight, it's possible you may have a thyroid or hormonal issue. In these situations, seek professional help from a licensed doctor in your area who may be able to do some tests and get to the root of the issue.

Do I need to work out to see results?

You don't need to work out to lose fat—it will just make things much easier. In terms of pure fat loss benefits, intense exercise can elevate your metabolism for hours after you work out, making your body burn extra calories all day long. Over time, as you build more lean muscle tissue, this tissue will also burn extra calories, even when you're just sitting on the couch. Lastly, exercise has many positive hormonal effects, particularly strength training, because it can trigger your body to release a lot of fat-burning hormones.

If you really can't exercise for some reason, it's possible to lose weight by just decreasing your food intake. However, you won't be able to eat as much, and you may you struggle to lose weight as you get leaner and leaner.

What happens if I go over my daily calories?

This happens all the time, especially in the beginning. It's best to just move on and try to get back on track with your next meal and commit to sticking to your plan the next day. Don't beat yourself up over it or try to starve yourself the next day to make up for it; it's just one meal.

If you go over by a lot or you want to enjoy a huge meal or social event, you can use the week to prepare. Look at your calories for the week. If your goal is to maintain a 3,500 calorie deficit per week by going under on calories by 500 each day, simply adjust the other days accordingly. You could increase your caloric deficit to 750 on the other six days, for example, giving you a lot more wiggle room on your big day.

This isn't necessary, of course, but if you're really dedicated and it'll make you feel better, it's fine to save a few hundred calories each day and use them later in the week to enjoy that fun social treat.

Should I adjust my macros in any way if I exercise that day?

No, that should be built in to the ratio we already developed. As long as you plan your meals so you get some of your carbs before and after your workouts, you should be fine. The extra need for calories on workout days should be included when you're figuring out your total calories.

Remember, carbs do more than just provide extra energy during your workout. They also help the recovery process when you're finished, even on days off. As long as you hit your macros each day and stay within the reasonable limits of your ratio, you should be just fine whether you're working out that day or not.

What if my food doesn't have a nutritional label?

Great question. Not all foods, especially fresh fruits and vegetables, have nutritional labels stuck to them. If you're not using a macro tracking app that automatically calculates all of this for you, it can be difficult to tell how many grams of protein a head of lettuce has.

Luckily, there are a lot of great resources online that track these kinds of things. While they might not always be completely accurate to the specific item you're holding (as they don't know the exact size of the apple or carrot stick), they can give a close enough approximation that it will fall within a reasonable margin of error for our macro ratio. Take a look in Appendix D: Additional Resources for more information.

APPENDIX B

Macro-Rich Foods

Carbohydrates

- Acai berries
- Apples
- Bananas
- Beans
- Beets
- Blackberries
- Black-eyed peas
- Blueberries
- Buckwheat
- Bulgur
- Cantaloupe
- Chickpeas
- Chips
- Corn
- Couscous
- Dates
- Energy bars
- Farro
- Grapefruit
- Grapes
- Green peas
- Lentils
- Lima beans
- Mango
- Millet
- Multigrain hot cereal
- Muffins
- Oatmeal
- Oranges
- Pancakes
- Parsnips
- Pasta
- Peaches
- Pears
- Pineapple
- Plums
- Potatoes
- Pretzels
- Pumpkin
- Quinoa
- Raisins
- Rice
- Sourdough bread
- Squash
- Strawberries
- Sweet potatoes
- Waffles
- Watermelon
- Whole-wheat bread
- Yams

Fat-Rich Foods

- Almonds
- Avocado
- Bacon
- Beef
- Butter
- Canola oil
- Cashews
- Chia seeds
- Cocoa butter
- Coconut
- Coconut oil
- Dark chocolate
- Duck
- Edamame
- Egg yolks
- Flaxseed
- Greek yogurt
- Heavy cream
- Hemp seed oil

- Macadamia nuts
- Mackerel
- Olive oil
- Olives
- Parmesan cheese
- Peanut butter
- Peanut oil
- Peanuts
- Pecans
- Pine nuts
- Pistachios
- Salmon
- Sardines
- Sour cream
- Soybeans
- Spirulina
- Sunflower seeds
- Tofu
- Tuna
- Walnuts
- Whole milk

Protein-Rich Foods

- 2% milk
- Amarath
- Anchovies
- Asparagus
- Beef
- Bone broth
- Broccoli
- Brussels sprouts
- Canned tuna
- Chicken
- Chorizo
- Cod
- Cottage cheese

- Eggs
- Grapefruit
- Greek yogurt
- Green beans
- Guava
- Halibut
- Hummus
- Kefir
- Kidney beans
- Lentils
- Mushrooms
- Nuts
- Passion fruit
- Pistachios
- Pomegranate
- Pork
- Pumpkin seeds
- Quinoa
- Rainbow trout
- Salmon
- Seitan
- Shrimp
- Soba noodles
- Soybeans
- Squash
- Spinach
- Spirulina
- Sun-dried tomatoes
- Swiss cheese
- Tempeh
- Tilapia
- Tofu
- Tuna
- Turkey
- Unsweetened cocoa powder
- Wheatgrass powder
- Whey protein

APPENDIX C

Glossary

Amino Acid
The building blocks of most of the cells in the human body.

ATP-PC System
The fast energy system. It can supply an intense burst of energy for around ten to twelve seconds.

Body Composition
The ratio of fat to lean tissue you carry.

Calorie
A measure of energy.

Carbohydrate
The body's preferred source of energy. These come from starchy foods such as potatoes and rice. They are the only nonessential macronutrient. Every gram of carbohydrate contains four calories.

Complex Carbohydrates
Carbohydrates that are broken down and digested slowly.

Conjugated Linoleic Acid (CLA)
A fatty acid associated with healthy body fat levels.

Fat
Stores energy, retains crucial vitamins, protects the organs, and encourages healthy skin and hair. Despite the shared name, this does not make you fat and is essential for your body. Each gram of fat contains nine calories.

Glucose
A simple sugar molecule.

Glycemic Index
Measures how fast carbs are digested. Carbs lower on the glycemic index will generally be higher in fiber and keep you feeling full longer.

Glycolytic System

The medium energy system. This powers your moderate-to-high intensity, short-duration activities, such as sprinting or lifting weights.

Macronutrient

Proteins, carbohydrates, and fats. They are essential to any good nutrition plan and supply the energy, fuel, and nutrients needed to live.

Micronutrient

The vitamins and minerals that allow your body to function at an optimal level.

Muscular Hypertrophy

The process of growing new muscle. It is the combined result of heavy resistance training and excess calorie intake.

Omega-3 Fatty Acids

One of two common omega fatty acids. It can increase mental functions, decrease the risk of cardiovascular disease, decrease inflammation and joint pain, and offers many more benefits.

Omega-6 Fatty Acids

One of two common omega fatty acids. It is common in processed and fried foods. Avoid when possible.

Oxidative System

The slow energy system. This provides a sustained release of energy for low-to-moderate activities such as long runs, swimming, or hiking.

Protein

Helps rebuild and repair damaged tissue and cells. This is essential for optimal health and body functioning. Every gram of protein contains four calories.

Saturated Fats

A decent kind of fat. You need some of these, but try to avoid them when possible.

Simple Carbohydrates

Carbohydrates that are broken down and digested quickly.

Trans Fats

The only truly bad fat. These have a negative effect on your cholesterol and heart health.

Unsaturated Fats

The best kind of fat. These have been shown to improve your good cholesterol and reduce your bad cholesterol.

APPENDIX D

Additional Resources

To download the bonus material for this book, including shopping lists, an up-to-date recommended supplement list, additional meal plans, a free workout program, and more, visit www.mattdustin.com/macronutrients. You can also find a contact form on this page to reach the author directly with any questions. If you want to look up nearly any supplement ingredient out there or find recommended supplements for specific health concerns, visit www .examine.com. Examine.com is the number one resource for all things nutrition and supplementation, providing completely unbiased and comprehensive scientific research reviews for just about anything related to supplementation.

Standard US/Metric Measurement Conversions

VOLUME CONVERSIONS

US Volume Measure	Metric Equivalent
⅛ teaspoon	0.5 milliliter
¼ teaspoon	1 milliliter
½ teaspoon	2 milliliters
1 teaspoon	5 milliliters
½ tablespoon	7 milliliters
1 tablespoon (3 teaspoons)	15 milliliters
2 tablespoons (1 fluid ounce)	30 milliliters
¼ cup (4 tablespoons)	60 milliliters
⅓ cup	90 milliliters
½ cup (4 fluid ounces)	125 milliliters
⅔ cup	160 milliliters
¾ cup (6 fluid ounces)	180 milliliters
1 cup (16 tablespoons)	250 milliliters
1 pint (2 cups)	500 milliliters
1 quart (4 cups)	1 liter (about)

WEIGHT CONVERSIONS

US Weight Measure	Metric Equivalent
½ ounce	15 grams
1 ounce	30 grams
2 ounces	60 grams
3 ounces	85 grams
¼ pound (4 ounces)	115 grams
½ pound (8 ounces)	225 grams
¾ pound (12 ounces)	340 grams
1 pound (16 ounces)	454 grams

OVEN TEMPERATURE CONVERSIONS

Degrees Fahrenheit	Degrees Celsius
200 degrees F	95 degrees C
250 degrees F	120 degrees C
275 degrees F	135 degrees C
300 degrees F	150 degrees C
325 degrees F	160 degrees C
350 degrees F	180 degrees C
375 degrees F	190 degrees C
400 degrees F	205 degrees C
425 degrees F	220 degrees C
450 degrees F	230 degrees C

BAKING PAN SIZES

American	Metric
8 x 1½ inch round baking pan	20 x 4 cm cake tin
9 x 1½ inch round baking pan	23 x 3.5 cm cake tin
11 x 7 x 1½ inch baking pan	28 x 18 x 4 cm baking tin
13 x 9 x 2 inch baking pan	30 x 20 x 5 cm baking tin
2 quart rectangular baking dish	30 x 20 x 3 cm baking tin
15 x 10 x 2 inch baking pan	30 x 25 x 2 cm baking tin (Swiss roll tin)
9 inch pie plate	22 x 4 or 23 x 4 cm pie plate
7 or 8 inch springform pan	18 or 20 cm springform or loose bottom cake tin
9 x 5 x 3 inch loaf pan	23 x 13 x 7 cm or 2 lb narrow loaf or pate tin
1½ quart casserole	1.5 liter casserole
2 quart casserole	2 liter casserole

Index